Patricia's Voice

Hope-Peace-Love

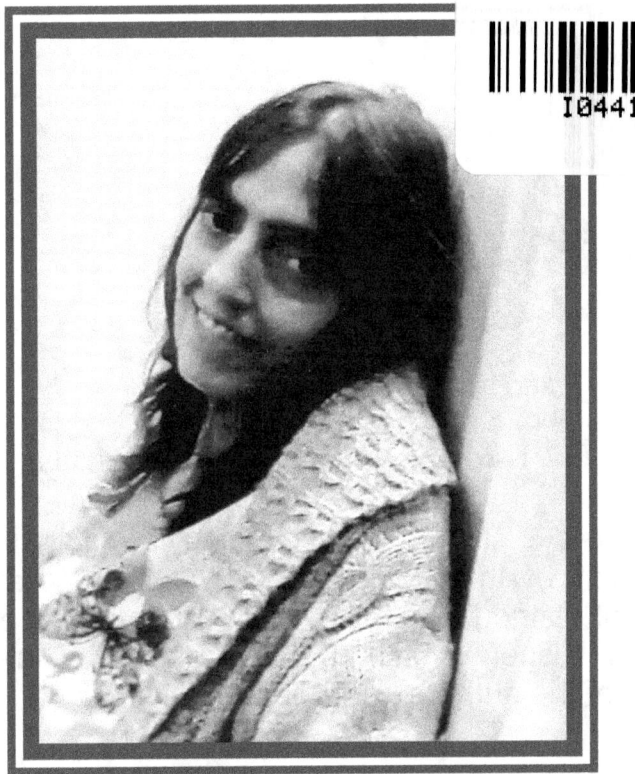

I0441274

A True Story

Eric **E. R**oberts

Author Eric E. Roberts

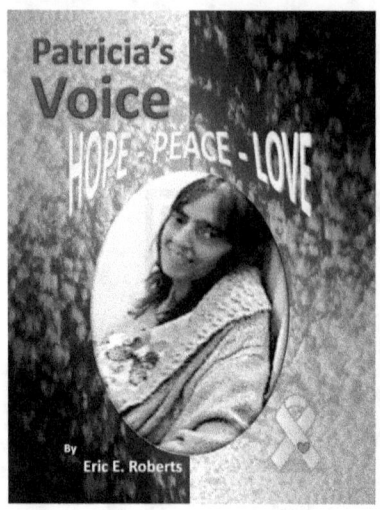

Patricia's Voice
Hope-Peace-Love

Cover Design by Danny Johnson
Interior Design by Danny Johnson
Author Photograph by Danny Johnson
Cover and Album Photographs by Eric E. Roberts - Author

Patricia's Voice
Hope-Peace-Love
ISBN-13:978-1535428651
ISBN-10:1535428651

This page intentionally reserved for Book Signing Events, Author's Autograph, Presentations and Gifting Options.

Dedication

I dedicate my first book (MFB) to **<u>Patricia Ann Fraley</u>**, my best Friend and Soulmate that anyone could ever ask for. I am so blessed that you came in to my life. Someone needed to be Patricia's Voice and I have the Devine Opportunity to be that Voice! Patricia, I got this!

I can only hope and pray this story will shine a light on the lack of communication in our healthcare industry.

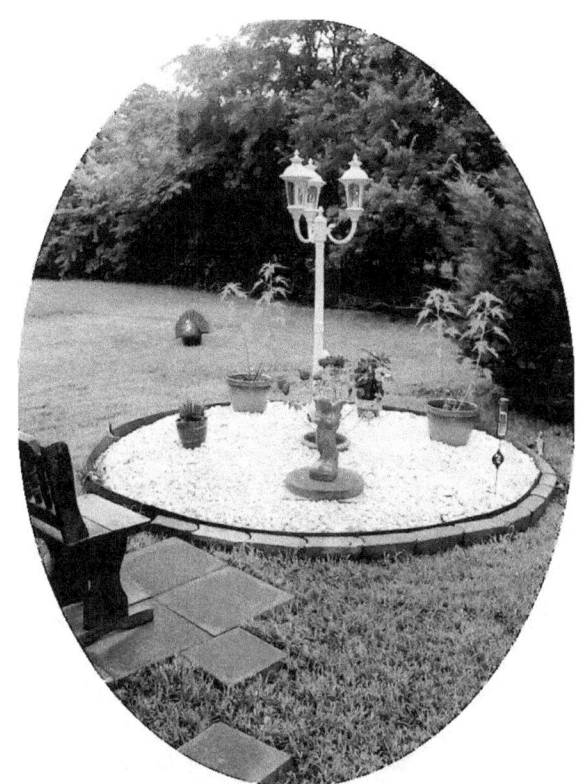

In Loving Memory
Of
Patricia Ann Fraley

Author Eric E. Roberts

08/23/2015

Dear Jesus,

It's 6:30 PM, Saturday evening. I am writing you this, to tell you, that I know the peace of God, which passeth all understanding. I hope I have told you enough how much I love you, Jesus. Thank you so much for your grace and I'm finding out more about my soul and how you said, guard your heart and your soul. Thanks for that. I am still working on my joy and with the help of the Holy Spirit, we got this! Thank you again for taking Patricia to be with you in heaven and every time you see Patricia say hi for me and please let her know the yard looks great and that she would be so proud of the girls and they are okay too. Let Patricia know she's all right in my book and that I love her! I got this.

Thank you Jesus!

Your Brother,

Eric

www.EricRoberts-Author.com

Acknowledgments

First I would like to thank our Lord and Savior, Jesus Christ and the Holy Spirit for having given me the strength to write this Book!

I also would like to thank all the Healthcare Givers from Hospice Plus. All of the staff did an outstanding job. God bless!

I also would like to give a, "Heartfelt Thank You," to all four of the Girls. Melinda, Katie, Kellie and Kristie, I know your mother is looking down from heaven and is so proud of all four of you. God bless!

Finally, a **Big Thanks** to my Editor, Best Friend and Brother in Christ, Danny Johnson and his Family. Thank you so much my Friend for the outstanding work you did on the Cover, Design, Editing, Technical Support and the encouraging words you gave me throughout this whole process. God bless!

www.EricRoberts-Author.com

Table of Contents

Foreword

My name is Eric Roberts. I have wanted to write a story for over 25 years. What took so long, you might ask? Well, a lot of it had to do with my lack of education and moving around from school to school, when I was an elementary student and throughout all of my school years.

All of the public schools that I attended were not able to provide adequate teaching for students with learning disadvantages. I literally learned how to write phrases and spell words by the way they sound to me. Most of my words are spelled wrong, but my spelling results in the same or slightly different pronunciations. The stories that I write, I keep in my journals and notebooks. I can understand my writings and spelling of words, but I have been reluctant to author any of my writings for fear of what others would say or think. Not anymore! I'm thanking God for, "Speech to Text

Technology." It has allowed me to read my stories aloud, while it listens and transcribes my stories, with acceptable spelling and grammar into a formatted document. I know the Holy Spirit is giving me the courage and desire to write this story. Patricia Ann Fraley is my inspiration.

I am writing my first book and dedicating it to Patricia, my true love, soul mate and best friend in the whole world. Patricia was my caring, loving and devoted Wife, a true gift from GOD, for nearly 21 years.

I am titling my book, "Patricia's Voice, Hope-Peace-Love." I believe and feel that this is a true story of a woman that fought the good fight, with GOD's Divine Grace and the love given to her from her LORD and Savior Jesus Christ, whom also sent the Holy Spirit to comfort her. GOD gave Patricia the Victory to overcome her alcohol addiction of 25 years in order to prepare her for the biggest fight of her life.

You see after 2½ years of being free of her alcohol addiction, the Doctor informed us in September 2014, that Patricia had stage "III-B Squamous Cell Cancer of the Cervix."

In her fight with cancer, Patricia grew very close to GOD and strengthened her faith and confirmed her salvation through our LORD and Savior, Jesus Christ.

GOD is always good to us and is always with us. This has proven to be true through the best of times and even the hardest trials and temptations of our lives. GOD cares for all of us. He knows us even before we were created. He knows just how we will complete our lives.

My hopes and prayers for "Patricia's Voice" are to reach as many people as possible and provide "Hope, Peace and Love."

On Sunday, May 24, 2015, God gave the final victory to Patricia. No more pain. No more tears. She is with our LORD. My Angel is watching over me.

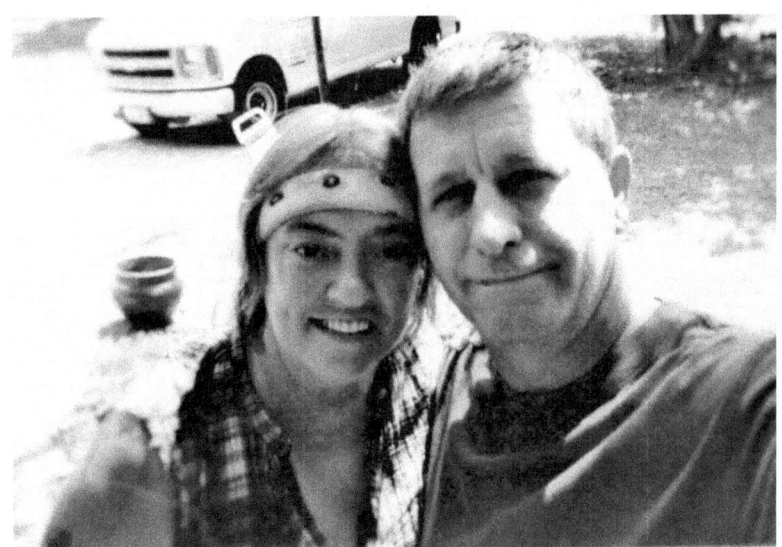

The search is over when soulmates connect

Patricia and I met each other on July 5th, 1994. I was a single father of a daughter that was 12 years old and Patricia had three girls, ages 3, 5 and 8 years old. I had a house full of girls.

You see, I was 30 years old and I wanted to be all I could be in the Army. I had just gotten back from being stationed in Omaha, Nebraska. After being up there for two years, I moved my daughter and me back to Texas, in the Dallas area, which is where I was raised up. Once you have lived in Texas, it seems to always call you back. When Patricia and I met, it was at a local karaoke bar and dance hall, where Patricia and I loved to dance. We put many miles on that dance floor.

I had been single for three years. My second wife kicked me out of the house after five years of marriage. That was back in 1990. I was thinking after 2 failed marriages I would just go and join the

Army at 30 years old. Hey, I did it and I was doing pretty well. I was really enjoying the single life and thought I would never settle down with another woman again. That was until I met Patricia and that changed everything. You see, I went to join the Army to be all I could be. I am so glad that I did, it helped prepare me for the next chapter of "Living with an Alcoholic." You will read that whole story in my next book. For now, I am going to pick up this story from three years ago.

We had just come out of fighting a "Whiskey Demon," for 17½ years and let me tell you, it took all the prayers and pleadings that I could muster, to try to get Patricia to stop drinking. **God love her!** Don't get me wrong! This story is not about Patricia's drinking. This story is about the good fight of a woman that got the "C-Word," as I believe Patricia and I had a true love that even the drinking could not tear us apart. I had to learn Patricia's every move in order to be keen on her likes and dislikes, as well as her pain and joys. It taught me to love her even more, even when it seemed impossible. I just wanted to be there for her and help her live and fight this alcohol demon.

On the day Patricia collapsed from the alcohol poisoning, she got so sick, that she could not fight it any longer. It was eating her liver up. It was a "Call to all Prayer Warriors moment." I hit my knees and cried out to God, "Please save Patricia!" The prayers really helped, even the Doctors were amazed, after running some more tests two days later, the test results came back more positive and the Doctor said her liver is okay. Patricia was getting another chance as long as she would stop drinking the alcohol. **I just know it was the prayers, because Patricia was getting another chance.** I was so relieved to get some good news. Well, fortunately, Patricia has some brain functions that made her forget she even drank alcohol. God does work in mysterious ways in all things. This is not really how I thought she would quit drinking, yet I was so relieved, that the alcohol demon was finally removed from her.

After almost 2 weeks in the hospital, it was time to get started on a whole new way of life. This is where the real story begins for "Patricia's Voice." I hope this story will help someone else in their journey.

Our youngest daughter had just moved out of the house a year earlier at 20 years old. Yippy! Kid free, just Patricia, me and Wally the dog! Patricia really struggled with a lot of little things at first, like standing, low strength, and her poor little mind on short-term memory. I was working as a plumber and fortunately, I had precious time to be able to work closer with Patricia. The money wasn't bad either. I got my strength through my prayers to Jesus. Patricia stopped asking for alcohol and I was so taken back by the sudden change of her thought process. It is like the memory of drinking was erased from her. It was nothing short of a miracle.

At first I just couldn't leave Patricia home alone. I was able to take her with me on some of my service calls. Patricia would bring a book to read or some crossword puzzles to do. She listened to the radio while I would be doing a job. I would go out to the van as much as I could, to check on Patricia and to let her know I'm almost finished and we'll be leaving soon. I sure enjoyed Patricia running around with me. She was such a joy, like a good friend, a very good buddy, if you know what I mean. We would drive through a hamburger place, pull over, then eat and talk. It was like getting to know the sober Patricia. That's when I started calling her Patricia. Before, it was just Trish. I was so proud of how Patricia Ann was adjusting, getting stronger and more independent.

Every chance we got, Patricia and I would do exercises. Some of them we would just make up as we went along. I went out and bought some weights and a stretch band. I even bought a treadmill to help her get stronger by walking on it.

Author Eric E. Roberts

Patricia has such a great will and attitude. We would often say things to each other for motivation like, "We got this!" or "We are in it to win it!" I love her so much and was so glad to see Patricia have a new chapter in her life without the alcohol. I would say oftentimes, "You are all right in my book!"

We had a new love and understanding about each other that we would call, "True Love." It even intensified even more, as if that is possible. After about four months, I believe her mind was getting a little sharper and clearer. Patricia said she felt like she was ready to go back to work. I was thinking it might be worth a try. You see before, "Breakfast," was out of the question and now three or four months later she is eating three square meals a day. That is great, eating good and getting healthier each day. All four girls were out on their own, doing their own thing.

We both are so very proud of all four of our girls. They would come over when they could to give their mother encouraging words. In a way, I felt that the girls blamed me for their mother getting so sick on the alcohol but I didn't know at the time if they understood the struggles their mother had with her drinking. Lord knows I tried to get Patricia to stop, but she just wanted to drink. I understand now why they felt the way they did, even when she got so swollen and started turning yellow in her eyes, I begged her to let me take her to the Doctor, the emergency room, or something. But, if you would have known Patricia, you'd know that she was so stubborn and hardheaded when it came to going and seeing a Doctor. Even one of the older girls came over with her husband and begged her mother to go to the Doctor. I told all the girls, I begged and pleaded so hard to get their mother to go get medical help, but no one can make her go. No matter how hard we pushed, Patricia just wouldn't go! The girls even went to the hospital to ask if I could get in trouble if I did not bring her into the emergency room. They even asked if the paramedics could come and get their mother and force her to go. They were told that Patricia would have to come in on her own, and that she would have to make that decision because she is an adult.

Two days later, Patricia got so sick it took our son in-law and me to carry her out to the truck because she was a little heavy. I drove her to the emergency room here in town. There was a lot going on around the hospital that morning. They had just locked the hospital down. Something about somebody got shot in downtown. We live in a small town. You can probably tell by now this is my first book. This is the most writing I have ever done at one time and this is a learning experience for me. I'm sure the editor will make it look good. Ok, I am going to move back to Patricia getting better.

Patricia wanted to do something productive. I guess it has been 4 ½ months now and we thought it would be nice for Patricia to work at a tree and grass farm. She could water, mow grass and trim the trees. Back when Patricia and I met, that is what she was doing. She did landscaping work, it's in her blood. That would be just the job for Patricia. I just happen to know a lady, Ms. C that owns a tree and grass farm right here in town, just a couple miles away. I was thinking I can take Patricia back and forth to work. She was now ready to start working again. Patricia got her shorts, favorite bandana and her cut off sleeveless shirt on. She was dressed for landscaping. I was proud of Patricia's eagerness to go back to work, so we went on out there to start work.

Patricia did not know that I went up there the day before and spoke with the owner of the company. I explained to her how Patricia was having a little trouble with her thinking sometimes and may get confused, but it would be good therapy for Patricia to get out of the house and do something she loves doing. That is to work outside. Just to be able to work with plants and be outside that was the ideal job for her. Ms. C said that she would keep an extra eye on Patricia and she would be happy to do what she could to help Patricia get stronger.

Well we got to the farm around 7:00 AM the next morning, ready to go to work. Patricia really looked happy while Ms. C showed Patricia all around the farm and showed her what plants to water. I sat in the office and visited with the owner for around an hour before I left just to make sure that Patricia was going to be okay. I went outside and told Patricia, "I love you! Have fun and call me if you need anything." It was hard to leave her there, but Patricia was so willing to work. I got back home, maybe one hour went by and the phone rang. Patricia was on the other end saying, "Please come get me I'm not ready to do this right now." I said, "Sure baby, I'll be right there in 10 minutes." Ms. C understood and told Patricia if she would ever like to come back and work, she was more than welcome to. Patricia felt so bad that maybe she had failed. I told her "No don't feel that way, when you are ready we will try again."

Patricia and I went home, to work on a new game plan.

We both knew one thing for sure. We love everything about our home. So we just threw ourselves into fixing up this old farmhouse. It was out in the country. We have a big long row of pine trees out front and a long driveway leading up to the house and beautiful crepe myrtle trees up the driveway. This old house was built back in 1958. Patricia and I have been living here for six years now and we really love it here.

When we found this house it was perfect timing. It was the perfect place for Patricia. I worked as much as I could to help Patricia build her confidence back up. We planted trees and kept busy mowing this place. It's almost an acre. Patricia loved mowing this whole place with a push mower. She loves mowing so much she would hardly ever let me push mow. I couldn't get the mower away from her! She said, "No way! This helps me think!"   She would fight you for the mower! God love her! Patricia and I had so much fun together, fixing this place up, landscaping, and painting the house. We put up a flagpole in the front yard. We even put up a white cast iron, 3 tier lamppost and ran electricity out to it, so it can shine each night. Even the landlord came by and said it looks so nice that his taxes were going to go up!   That's so funny! I will say, "It was a lot of work."

What a partnership! We were growing closer and closer. We were soul mates. We both were good for each other. I believe God had something to do with it! We have been together up to this point in time for 17½ years. This would make a great love story....... Well, it is that too! We would set out front at our picnic table and just admire how this place was looking. The hard work is paying off. Patricia was so happy and pleasant. A side of Patricia that I know I am blessed to know. I think she was recognizing the battle she had just fought. We made the Fourth of July, the anniversary of the day

Patricia stopped drinking. I got her an anniversary card for that first year and gave it to her. Patricia cried. I even heard her cry out to God and thank him for delivering her from that addiction. She was so thankful and she looked at me with the most loving look and said, "Thank you Eric. You are the love of my life." I was so thankful to God that Patricia was over that fight too. God love her!

Patricia is the love of my life. Sometimes I would call her, "Love Muffin" or "My Sunshine." Each time we would talk on the phone, I would tell her, "I'm heading to another service call and I will see you later." She would always say, "Be careful!" and I would say, "Always!" That's how our conversations would end. Patricia would always tell me, that if she just had a small pickup she would put a lawnmower in the back of it and start her own mowing and landscaping business. We were able to save up just enough money to pay cash for a 1998 Dodge Dakota pickup. It is pretty nice. It is silver. I felt it would be a nice and safe reliable truck for her to work out of. Patricia was so excited when I brought it home.

I was so happy to see Patricia's response over it. I love this woman. That's how she makes me feel every day. I was given this opportunity to get to know the most caring, giving, and loving woman I have ever met. I cannot say enough. I tried to encourage Patricia to drive the truck but she was not quite ready yet. We called it her truck and I told Patricia it will be right there in the driveway just in case you are ever ready to drive it. I think it just being in the driveway and able to see it gave Patricia even more confidence. Plus, when I'm out working in my work van, it was good that the truck was there in the driveway for security reasons, being out in the country and all. Patricia loves this place so much. The house is small and easy to keep up. It felt so in the country and it also helps keep Patricia busy.

By this time, 2 more years had gone by. We were on Patricia's second anniversary of being alcohol free. Patricia was so proud of herself. Our 19th year anniversary falls on July 5. We had been there now eight years at this rent house. Just for Patricia, I built something that she has always wanted, a deck down the whole front of the house. It is over 30 feet long and 5 ft. wide with a tin roof.

Patricia and I love spending time out there when it rained, we would listen to it hit the tin roof. We put white rock around the lamppost out front. It's about 15 ft. around and it looks pretty cool. I put some pictures in the back of this book, so you too can enjoy the scenery. It's pretty to look at. "No worries!" she would say. I just got a joy sitting out front and watching her mow the lawn. I know it's nothing short of a miracle that Patricia had come this far. I guess you can say Patricia had the eye of the Tiger.

The improvements Patricia had made to that point were outstanding. Do I need to say more? It was even nice to see the girls starting to come around more to visit. They could even see their mother becoming so peaceful and start to enjoy where she's at in her life. They were so glad to see their mother had not had a drink in just over two years. We all were so proud of Patricia. The girls all got together and made a card. That was so sweet of them! Then they gave it to their mother, and it read like this:

"To: Mommy dearest, from your favorite daughters. Happy Mother's Day! We are so proud of you and how far you have come in the last year. Keep up the amazing work! You are the most amazing Mom anyone could ask for. For we wouldn't be who we are without you! You taught us how to be strong and always take up for ourselves. You taught us to keep our heads up and everything will be okay. We wouldn't trade you for the universe. Thanks for being the most awesome mom in the world!

Always your daughter's!

Kristie, Katie, Kellie, and Melinda."

Living out here in this wonderful country house with this entire yard to keep up was just what the doctor ordered for Patricia. Patricia loves this house and she keeps it up so nice and clean. She would often say this place is, "Home Sweet Home." I just could not wait to get off work and rushed home to the love of my life and my friend. We would say, "This is country living at its finest! No worries! We got this old place looking pretty good and it is all worth it."

One day I came home from work and Patricia was complaining of her lower back hurting. She blamed it on the leg exercises she was doing. After two weeks of her complaining about her back pain, Patricia also seemed to be getting weaker. I asked Patricia if she would like me to take her to see the doctor. Patricia said no, she was just going to change her exercise routine for now and she would start drinking some protein shakes.

Three weeks after that, she was having trouble with her bowel movements for almost a week. She seemed to be getting weaker and having trouble with walking. I finally said "Love Muffin, something is just not right here. I am taking you to the Hospital Emergency Room." I picked Patricia up and carried her to the truck.

The hospital is only 2 miles away. I went in and grabbed a wheelchair and got her in as fast as I could. I called one of the girls on the cell phone to let her know that I have their mother at the hospital, and please call the other girls and let them know what is going on. They took Patricia right into the emergency room ran some blood tests. Within 15 minutes the results came back that her kidneys were failing. They were going to rush Patricia to the main hospital in Dallas, because they had a Kidney Specialist working out of that hospital. She would be going by ambulance and I could meet them there and there was no time to waste. I told Patricia I would be there when she arrived at the hospital in Dallas. It's about an hour away from here.

I called the girls on the way to let them know that the ambulance was taking their mother to the Dallas hospital. It looks like her kidneys were bad, and we would see the girls there. I was praying to Jesus all the way to Dallas, "God please take care of Patricia and give me strength to do the right thing and to say the right things, please help Patricia through this." Lord knows we had just fought one battle. I was hoping it was just a bad diagnosis and this will work out with God's help.

I really started to lean on Jesus. I guess I got it from my mama. My Mother did raise me to know that God is there if we ever need to call upon him. Thanks to God for Sunday school where we learned to sing songs like the old-time favorites. You never forget the saying, "Jesus loves me yes I know. For the Bible tells me so." I will say this again, "All thanks be to GOD!" We can go to him in prayer to ask for strength. Let me tell you something, if you or someone you know has kidney problems, you already know you get really sick. I always knew that the kidneys were important. But to find out like this! I was so scared for Patricia and knowing she was so confused. It hurt me so much to see this happening to her. Patricia is such a sweet lady.

They took her right in at the Dallas hospital and started running more tests and x-rays. The girls started arriving to the hospital. Patricia was so out of it. The Kidney Doctor came in after reviewing the test that they ran. He said that Patricia may have to go on kidney dialysis. She was so sick that they were going to have to give her a blood transfusion. They had Patricia in ICU. They asked me to leave the room and to go down the hall and wait in the waiting area until they got the IV started for the blood transfusion. It was breaking my heart. I could hear Patricia crying out in pain, it was so sad. I just wanted to run in there and tell them to stop. I thought, oh GOD! Patricia and I do not even like hospitals and here Patricia is, going through all this.

The first five hours was a nightmare, if you can understand. Like if it was your

Four-year-old child crying out for you to come save them. I will never forget it. From the pain or the medication Patricia was on she was going into a comatose state, not very aware. By this time 2 of the girls were arriving and Patricia's older sister was just arriving too. The hospital ICU said we would have to wait a while until Patricia was stable before they would let anyone else go back.

I could feel the tension right away. It seems like everyone wanted to put the blame on me, the oldest sister says right off, "Patricia had to be real sick for a long time. What took you so long to get her into the hospital?" I explained to her, "For about three weeks I tried to get Patricia to go in to see a doctor for her lower back pain that she was having." I told her, "If you know Patricia, it is so hard to get her to go see a doctor." Even after saying that, I can still feel the tension. I told myself that I need not let that cloud my thinking. My most concern at that time was to find out what was going on with Patricia. Thinking she's going to need my help more than ever now. We were going to navigate through this and we were going to get it fixed.

My sweet love was fighting with all she has and I could see it in her face. I felt so helpless. I just wanted to know what was next. I spoke with each doctor and each R.N. that had any questions about Patricia's health. I guess I know her best. After 19 years and six months together, you get to know your partner pretty darn good. You have to become the "Voice" of your loved one. I just knew right from the start, I was going to do everything in my ability and the strength from God to help Patricia. I know she would do the same for me. That's unconditional love. They were saying they needed more tests. Patricia's blood was all out of whack. I really felt that the family had good intentions for their behavior. I understood their great concern for their mother. I could feel something was going on behind the scenes. Deep inside I still know it.

At first, the girls and some of the family wanted to take over Patricia's healthcare. They even had gone as far as telling the hospital staff that we were not even legally married. That maybe it was my fault Patricia is this sick. They were even asking if they could take over signing for medical procedures that needed to be performed on their mother's behalf. Blaming me started working on me, at first. I was hurt.

I called my older sister for some counseling. I felt alone at first, I needed a new look on the matter. My sister gave me some good advice saying that I would have to be the adult here and it's understandable how the girls were acting. Patricia is their mother, and she would feel the same way if it was her mother, you are just the stepdad. My sister said to me, "Just let them know that you love their mother and you are there for the same reason they are, to see Patricia get better."

She told me you need to get them all together and tell them if it was not for you and your patience they probably would not have their mother this long. You stayed with her this long and not to blame you for what Patricia has gone through to get herself here the last 20 years. "By golly, you been there for her up to now and you sure are there now for her." Now, I am glad that I called my sister. I needed to get a word from someone on the outside. She knows what I went through and she was very helpful. I understand the tensions and emotions were running high at the time we all were just getting over the liver incident from 2 ½ years ago.

Well finally, they let us all go back into ICU where Patricia was. I was hoping so much that she would wake up so the girls could get her story of what got us here now. I feel that Patricia would not have liked how the girls were acting towards me. I was not the enemy. I was pretty concerned that if Patricia does wake up, how would her thinking be, and her memory? How clear is her mind going to be so she can explain to the girls there is nothing that I was doing?

We were all in the room, standing around the bed, when all of a sudden Patricia opened her eyes and smiled and started joking. She looked around the room and knew everybody's name. I was so glad to see how clear Patricia's mind was in her memory. I was so worried about that. After seeing that, I went down to the truck in the underground parking garage to the hospital and turned on some music. I think the song was "Royal," and started doing the happy dance.

See, the girls did not live with Patricia and we had a great love. The way I was looking at it we were happy and things are looking good. This was much unexpected for us. I think maybe just a little bit in their thinking, they thought it has something to do with the drinking. I know I was there every day. Patricia had not touched a drop of liquor in over 2 ½ years. That's outstanding to me.

Later on in the evening Patricia's oldest daughter was sitting in the room, it was just Kellie and I, Patricia was sleeping. I explained to Kellie that I could feel maybe something was going on in the background. With them wanting to take Patricia away from me, but I told her you need to understand the love that me and your mother share is a true love. Her mother felt the same way towards me too and if she were more awake and clear right now, she would tell her the same thing. She told me, "You are telling me this, because I am the most gullible." I told Kellie, "No, I am telling you this because I think you are very wise and have a good head on your shoulders. You know that coming between your mother and I would not be good for her at all." I really felt that she was starting to get it now. I was there for the good and just how much I care for her mother.

For the first three nights I stayed right there in the room with Patricia. The hospital brought in a chair that I could lay on and sleep there in the ICU. I was going to watch over Patricia like a hawk, that is just who I am. I will have to say that all the R.N.'s and Doctors working in ICU were doing an outstanding job of trying to get Patricia stable, but I do have a few concerns I would like to mention.

One evening, one of the R.N.'s told Patricia if she did not calm down that your husband would have to leave the room and she would be all by herself. What is that about? Another thing is the blood transfusion, the IV that was in Patricia`s arm was leaking all over a pillow that she had her arm laying on. When the next R.N. came into the room, I pointed it out and mentioned that it was leaking. The R.N. told me he would be back around a little bit later to change it out and fix it. I guess it was four hours later when the ICU R.N. finally came in and cleaned it up and redid the IV in Patricia's arm.

I started noticing that the nurses were working from 7 AM to 7 PM. That is a long shift, sometimes longer. When you figure that they come in an hour before the shift starts, and sometimes leaves an hour after their shift ends. Going over medical charts with the other staff I can see it in their faces. I understand they work their butts off. I think that is a lot of hours for one person to have to work. I don't care who you are, working that long of a shift just sets yourself up to make mistakes. Some could be big. Well, that was one of my first observations of the medical field. I was beginning to learn that communication is very important right from the start.

X-Ray results came back. Patricia has a Tumour!

Well the CAT Scan and X-ray results came back telling us that it looked like Patricia has a tumor that is pushing on her kidneys and her lower back. That is starting to explain what was causing the lower back pain and not having good bowel movements for almost 2 weeks. They told us, in order to give Patricia some relief on her kidneys, they will have to take her down to the oncology and install nephrostomy tubes into her kidneys.

By this time, I could feel that the tension between the girls and Patricia's Sisters was easing up a bit. There was still a little bit of tension. I just put it in God's hands for now. The girls want to sign a release form for the doctor to work on her nephrostomy tubes. I just let that go, getting the treatment was the most important thing at this time, not bickering over who was going to sign papers. This situation had us all on pins and needles. The procedure went pretty good, it helped get some of that poison out of Patricia's kidneys so she can start thinking clear. After being in ICU for five days, they were talking about moving Patricia up to her own room upon the sixth floor.

I am still hoping that maybe something that I am sharing in this book will help shine a little light on the healthcare industry, the good and the bad. Don't forget I am just a plumber and was learning for the first time, the highs and the lows. This story is about "Patricia's Voice," a "Voice" maybe to someone that is having the fight of their lives, and a time to pull out your total faith in Jesus.

I know Patricia was confused and there was so much going on, but I was sure to let her know that I am right here. I am going to hold your hand and we are going to go through this together no matter what. I hope I have expressed enough to this point how much I love this woman. I just had to get that in there.

Back to the healthcare industry! Let me tell you if someone you love, Lord forbid that ever happens, just be mindful of how the R.N.'s, Doctors, Specialists, and anyone involved with the care of your loved one. Especially if they cannot make decisions on their own for whatever reason, being unconscious, or confused to some kind of mental status. I am sure there are a lot more reasons. What was good for Patricia and I, is that we have been with each other for over 17 years knowing what each other's likes and don't likes are and so much more. We come to find out that we were in the same hospital even in ICU at the same time that there was the Ebola patient.

We all were relieved when they brought Patricia up to her own room. It was better, a little more privacy and quieter. Patricia's mind seems to be getting clearer from all the toxins that were removed from her body. The hospital brought in a fold out bed so I could stay in the room with Patricia. I know Patricia was so sick. It was so much of a relief that her mind was getting clear.

Now it was going into the second week of being in the hospital. The girls were so happy to see their mother getting more responsive. Patricia was being her funny self a little more. She would joke with the doctors, the R.N.'s, and anyone she could make laugh. Patricia has the greatest personality. What a great spirit, with all that was going on, not to mention all the blood tests. It seemed like they were drawing blood every four hours, I would stay with Patricia as much as possible. I made a few service calls to make money to keep the lights on at the house.

On the days I would have to work, one of the girls would stay with their mother. God bless them for that. We tried our best to make sure that a family member stayed with Patricia. I was learning a lot more about texting on the telephone. On days when I would be out working the girls and I would text back and forth if we had some different news on Patricia's test results.

After three weeks in the hospital, I was sure getting homesick. After learning more about Patricia's diagnosis, running a CAT scan, and taking a biopsy of the tumor, the results came back that Patricia has Stage 3 Cancer of the Cervix. I would have never thought that Patricia would have cancer. It struck all of us so hard. We started making plans on getting Patricia treatment for her cancer. The doctor said with Patricia having stage III, she would need chemo treatment. I know that would be hard to pay for but we would manage somehow. Patricia was not working, so no insurance there. I had no insurance either.

We found out it is hard to get insurance when you have a pre-existing illness and we were not very big fans of Obama care. Being self-employed, my taxes needed to be brought up to date. We looked into the Medicaid system. We got a social worker from the hospital to take the case to see what they could do about getting Patricia some coverage. It was almost our only option at the time.

After a month, the hospital was ready to send Patricia home. Believe me, Patricia Ann was ready. Patricia and I are a lot of a like when it comes to being at home, that is what we loved the most at this time in our lives, and we are what you would call, "Home Bodies." The hospital gave us a lot of instructions on the medication. There were about five different medications Patricia had to take each day and a list of follow-up appointments to see three different specialists, one each for kidney, oncologist, and radiation. Included also was a list of the do's and don'ts.

This was around 9:15 AM, the first week in October 2014. We scheduled an appointment with kidney doctor over in Dallas. Patricia's kidney count was getting better. That was good news. Then we scheduled an appointment with the doctor that did the biopsy on the tumor.

Dr. "O" told us that Patricia would have a good chance if she could get started right away on chemo treatments. It might help fight the cancer off and help with the leg pain from the tumor pressing on the sciatic nerve in her leg. He told us there was a place closer to our home we could go to get treatment and explained that Patricia would have to go each day for six weeks and it doesn't hurt. Two of the girls were there that day when we spoke with Dr. "O." He gave us a prescription for pain, not for us but for Patricia, that is. I had gone out and bought Patricia a wheelchair to get her around to her appointments. So glad I did, we like easy.

At home Patricia started using her walker to get around the house more to hang her nephrostomy tube bag on. She was more confident doing it that way. I was keeping in contact with the other clinic, the one Dr. "O" recommended us too. I explained to them, we were waiting to hear back from Medicaid for payment. We sure wanted to get some kind of treatment started. When you have no insurance, nobody will talk to you. You see, when we left the hospital, their job was only to get Patricia stable. There was really no other treatment they could do for her. It was going to have to come from the outside.

We had been sitting at home now for two weeks. No treatment started yet. It was going almost 3 weeks now. I even called up to the other clinic and was willing to pay $600 just for consultation. I was willing to do that, just to get more information and try to get something started for Patricia, maybe even some chemo treatments. Still, even that was not going to get treatment started. The receptionist at the clinic told me I would have to pay cash. I got us an appointment one week from today. It just seems like there was just so much delay. Patricia and I not having insurance caught us so off guard. God love her.

Patricia's 2 older sisters came over to the house to visit one afternoon. They were asking why is there no treatment started yet? I explained to Sharon and Karen that we were waiting on Medicaid and believe me, we wanted to get treatment started too. Karen and Sharon gave us this idea to go to Parkland Hospital in Dallas that they would take Patricia right in and treat her. I was ready to try anything to get Patricia some kind of treatment started right away. I knew Patricia needs chemo if we want to fight this cancer as early as possible. Patricia had a real nice visit with her sisters and after us talking about it, Patricia and I decided we would give it a try and go the next day.

The next morning, I laid out Patricia some clothes on the couch and was going to go to the store and get us breakfast. I think it was Whataburger. Patricia loves her Whataburger biscuits, gravy, eggs, and sausage, sounds good! I told Patricia as soon as I get back I would help her get dressed and we would go to Parkland and see if we can get right in. When I got back with the breakfast Patricia was already dressed. She was ready to go. I loaded up the wheelchair onto the truck, a bag with bottled water, and a list of all of her medication with all the paperwork we have from the Dallas hospital and off we went.

We got there early, it was around 8 o'clock and the lobby was packed, Patricia was doing great. She was setting up there in her little wheelchair like a little trooper just waiting for them to call her name.

It was about 20 minutes, faster than I thought it was going to be. They take Patricia back into this little room to take her vital signs, take her blood pressure and temperature. We explained to that technician how we were at the Dallas hospital and Patricia needed chemo treatments for her cancerous tumor. We had no insurance and the most important thing right now is, what we can do about getting chemo treatments.

After about 10 minutes, they made us wait longer out in the waiting area for the next stage. They called us back into another area took Patricia's blood pressure again after a couple more questions and sent us down to another area. They asked us a few more questions and had us sign a couple or three different papers. All this time Patricia is still sitting in her wheelchair.

It was almost 3 ½ hours, I know Patricia was getting frustrated and it was very uncomfortable for her too. I kept trying to encourage her and telling her that maybe now we can get some treatments, just hang in there just a little bit longer. Next thing you know, Patricia and I were down in another area of the hospital sitting in the hallway. There must have been 30 people sitting in the hallway. Patients were waiting in chairs, standing, and sitting in wheelchairs. It was a sight to see. I know Patricia was so uncomfortable, she really could not stand very long. Patricia was weak in her legs. God love her. I finally went over to the counter at the nurses' station and explain how Patricia was very uncomfortable. Maybe there was some where she could lay down. The lady behind the counter kind of snickered and said there is no place to lie down. Maybe if we were over at the new hospital there would be.

Finally, I stopped one of the doctors in the hallway and explain to him what was going on. I explained to the doctor that we already know Patricia has a tumor and we also know that it's at Stage III Cancer and Patricia needs Chemo Treatments. What can we do to get to that stage of not having to go through all these other ones to get to that point? Now something is happening, the Dr. had one of the aides' push Patricia around to the women's clinic on the other side of the hospital. That was about 5 ½ hours wasted.

They take Patricia back and put her in a room. Believe me, I stayed with her this whole time I was not going to let her out of my sight. They took her blood pressure again, her temperature, her vital signs, asked more questions, and brought in some paperwork.

Finally, Patricia looks up at me and says please, please, take me home. I can't take this anymore. I guess all the encouraging words were running pretty thin. I can understand how Patricia feels, even the doctors and nurses try to talk Patricia into staying but all she wanted to do was go home. I don't blame her. I am pretty worn out myself by this time. You know, we went back home. I know Patricia's sisters meant well, and we did give it our best try but the hospitals are not like the way they use to be 30 years ago. It is just too busy, especially for the condition Patricia was in at that time.

Patricia's pain pill medication was running very low, so I called the clinic of Dr. "O," the last doctor she had seen at the Dallas hospital. The secretary over the phone told me that they do not like writing prescriptions for the pain medication on patients that are no longer being seen. They would do it this time, but I would have to go to the Plano hospital. The doctor was working out the Plano hospital that day.

After breakfast that morning, I put Patricia some lunch on the coffee table in front of the couch and told her I will be right back. I am going to Plano to pick up your pain prescription, so I can get back and pick it up at the pharmacy here in town. It was a little over an hour drive over to the hospital in Plano. I believe I prayed all the way to the hospital asking God to please help me find some way to get Patricia started on some treatment. It was going on three weeks now.

After I got there, I found my way to the nurses' station at the clinic in the hospital to pick up the prescription. I asked the lady behind the counter, "Do you have a prescription for Patricia for me to pick up?" Oh boy, here came the tears right there in front of the secretary behind the counter. I explained to her, "Is there anybody here I can talk to, my wife is at home dying of cancer, we have no insurance, and we have nowhere to turn? Is there a financial counselor here that I can speak with?"

She directed me back to the counselor's office. I went back there to speak with her. I explained to her how Patricia was very sick and running a 102 temp. How we had been to the Dallas hospital, but all they could do was to stabilize Patricia, and send her home. How we have no insurance and no way to pay for chemo treatments. We felt so stuck and I did not know what to do. We even talked about indigent care. That is for when you have no insurance or you are homeless and the government will pay for your treatments. I tell you the lady there was so nice! She felt so bad that we were having this situation. I am going to give her great credit for the idea that she was about to give me.

She told me to go home, get your wife, and take her back to the hospital in Dallas where you were all at before. The doctors know Patricia there. Plus, her records are there and tell them to please treat your wife. She needs help and she needs it now. I thanked her, shook her hand, and left out of there with some great hope. I was praising God all the way home for the great information. It was an idea that I would have not thought about on my own. I know it was the Holy Spirit that guided me to ask those questions.

I went back to the house first before I was going to go pick up the prescription at the pharmacy. Patricia's leg pain seems to be worse and her fever is getting up there. I told Patricia lets go back to the Dallas hospital and let them treat you.

We need their help!

Patricia got dressed, I carried her to the truck, and off we went. Glad we did. We went right in to the emergency room. All her records were on the computer, all the doctors, and all her medication too. Patricia's temperature was rising over 102 and a lot of leg pain from the tumor pushing on her sciatic nerve in her right leg. The hospital ran all kinds of blood test. They came back. Patricia had a bad infection in her bladder and started giving her antibiotics right away.

I know we did the right thing. It was a big load off my shoulder just knowing Patricia was getting treatment from one of the best hospitals in Texas with great doctors and staff. I do know they need to work on their communication skills. You really don't know how important it is for the person that brings someone to the hospital to be the voice of that person if they are unable to speak or communicate their needs. I already made up my mind that I was going to be there for Patricia and help anyway I could to be her voice. To make sure that she had all her needs met to the best of my ability. I know she would do the same for me. I feel it was my job to be as positive as I can, no matter what. If you give positive out, you get positive back, Patricia and I both felt that way to all the Doctors, the R.N.'s, and even Housekeeping.

We treated everyone we met like that. I know I am just a plumber, but I am very observant, taking what I have learned from the first time Patricia and I were up here at the hospital. Even the little things like knowing how to order food for Patricia from the cafeteria menu, where the snack machines are, how to run the remote on the TV in her room, getting IVs, blood tests.   Even getting the right color hospital gown, the yellow one is for fall risk.   I even started a journal to write things down. I was observing the policies and procedures of the hospital staff.   It was a learning moment, watching with an open mind.

The hospital had to call in the center for disease control to find out what kind of infection was in Patricia's bladder and what kind of antibiotics to make up to fight the infection. That went on for weeks and then they finally got it under control. That was a relief for all of us. Thank God for that, God love her.

The doctor came in and told us that Patricia would be going down to radiation. She would be getting the doctor of radiology of oncology to look at her case. I sure wanted to be there to hear what they had to say about shrinking that tumor with radiation. When they came to get Patricia to push her over to the other side of the hospital, I was right there with her talking to her, encouraging Patricia, being positive, and even joking with the aid that was pushing Patricia down the hallway. It was a long hallway, two or three to be exact, and even a couple of elevator rides.

While Patricia and I were waiting in the room for the doctor of radiology to come in and meet us, we were talking of how great it is that she was getting treatment. I could see in her eyes the great hope. I think that comes from the piece of knowledge knowing that Jesus and both of us were talking about how God is in control. I know she was happy knowing that this radiation was supposed to help with the pain.

The doctor came in to talk with us. Patricia was lying on the bed that they brought her over on. The doctor that was speaking with us is a professor of radiology. He really knows just his field of study. He also had the best bedside manner of any of the doctors we have met so far. This doctor gave us very helpful information about what was going on inside of Patricia and with this tumor. He showed us x-rays that the hospital had taken earlier over a month or more ago. The Dr. explained how they were going to target that spot on the tumor that was pushing on the nerve in Patricia's leg. He also explained to us how they were going to take an x-ray picture of the target area of the tumor and draw a target on her stomach. Then they would shoot the radiation and that should help shrink the tumor back a little, Patricia and I was both so relieved. We felt a lot more informed about her tumor. We were fighting the tumor not cancer. Cancer was not in our vocabulary. That was not our focus at that moment.

They took Patricia back and took an x-ray, drew on her stomach a target, just like the doctor told us they were going to do. It was in dark ink, we both laughed at the way it looked. The technician says gave them 10 to 15 minutes to study the x-ray and then they would come back and get Patricia to give her the radiation treatment.

The radiation doctor came back in the room while we were waiting for the technician to come get Patricia. The doctor explained to us how the radiation would not hurt and how this is a new way of giving radiation to the target spot, but it would take about three days to notice the difference. This would help to shrink the tumor off of the nerve and Patricia's appetite would come back, but there will be diarrhea for maybe a week. Patricia laughed and said, "I can live with that, let's do this." We both were so happy that it was going to help get rid of the pain in her leg. Maybe even kill some of the cancer cells and give us more time to get funding for some chemo treatment.

When they came to pick up Patricia to take her back for her radiation treatment, I told the nurse I was going to step outside for a minute. I told Patricia I would be right here waiting for her to come back out. While I was sitting outside I prayed to God that this would help Patricia and thanking him for a great doctor that was very caring and concerning. It was not even 15 minutes later the nurse came out and told me they were done. I was thinking that was fast and easy. When we got back to Patricia's hospital room, Patricia was so hungry and ready to eat.

The next day the doctor that sent Patricia home the first time, did the biopsy of the tumor and said it was stage III, came into Patricia's room. He told us you do know that she has stage III cancer and maybe stage 4 by now and that it is in her bones. I said, "What? The bone......? No one has said anything about bone before." The Dr. said he would have to check into that, maybe he had miss read it.

The nurse came back into the room three hours later and told us that the doctor said he wants to take a biopsy of Patricia's bone on her lower spine and that the procedure would be the following day.

I am thinking this doctor needs to get it together the whole hospital has a communication problem. I even had to point out to the head nurse that Patricia has been here for a week now and she still hasn't had someone put a yellow gown on her to let everyone know that the patient is a fall risk and has trouble standing on their own. I told everyone I could when Patricia came in the first time.

This time Patricia is having trouble with her thinking, her memory, she was weak in the legs having trouble standing, and walking, and that she is a fall risk. I even tried to write in my journal each day to help me keep up with remembering all that was happening this time in the hospital.

This was a learning experience for me. Who would have ever thought I would be writing in a journal. I did this because I wanted to be of some help, to make things better for the next patient that comes into the hospital. You might say constructive criticism, even taking pictures from my cell phone. I was learning more and more each day and was observing what the nurses were more into, the diagnosis of the patient and what was on the computer screen. They were not so much worried about what the mental health of the patient is. Technology is a great tool but we are losing one on one with the patient by relying more on technology. That's ok but we need to work with both at the same time.

www.EricRoberts-Author.com

I am Grateful to be Patricia's Voice

I'm so glad I could be there to be Patricia's voice. I know her like the back of my hand. Each time a nurse would come into the room pushing the computer cart around with the patient's information on it. Like medication name, diagnosis, and what meds are due. I feel that along with that should be footnotes on the patient's mental strengths and weaknesses. Are their concerns being met? Are they listening to the family members or the person who brings the other person into the hospital? They need more open dialogue and better communication. I feel that a lot more could be done around that topic, but for now I will leave that to the professionals.

The next morning the technician came in early. It was around 7 AM and told us that Patricia was scheduled to go down to the OR and get her nephrostomy tubing changed out and they were going to do the bone biopsy on Patricia at the same time. They told us that Patricia was not allowed to eat or drink anything until after the procedure. I know it was so hard on Patricia being hungry and thirsty. Oh Lord and the diarrhea had started just like the doctor told us down in radiation. When 10:30 came around, we had not heard from anyone when they would be coming to take Patricia down to her procedure. I went out to the nurses' station and asked if they heard anything? All they could tell me is it would be anytime now. I went back and sat with Patricia and just held her hand trying to comfort her to let her know they said any minute now, they would be coming in to get you.

Four O 'clock came and we were still waiting. By this time Patricia was pretty hungry. Patricia had not eaten since the day before and she was asking for a drink of water. We only gave Patricia little sips. God love her. Patricia probably started to think she was being punished or something. A thought even crossed my mind that maybe by not having insurance and no money they may have bumped Patricia down the line a little further. I was just saying, but I let it go.

At 5:30 PM, I went back out to the nurse's station and asked to speak with the head nurse. They told me they would send her down to Patricia's room as soon as possible. When the head nurse came down, I went out into the hallway to speak with her and asked her what could be taking so long. Patricia is hungry, thirsty, and becoming anxious. She told me they were busy down there.

Then it was 8 PM when they came and got Patricia. I let the head nurse know about it. She just tells me again that they were just busy. Then I told the head nurse I can understand that but someone should have come in to let us know they are busy. Tell us it is going to be a while that way we could have played checkers or cards, sang songs, something, not just waiting and waiting thinking they are coming any minute.

We got down to the OR and the OR Nurse picked up the chart they sent Patricia with and says I do not think this is you, your name is not Tyesha. We all laughed at that. I am telling you that had a lot to do with communication. The OR nurse called up to Patricia's floor and asked if they would bring the correct medical chart down to the OR. The doctor told me it would be about two hours before they would bring Patricia back up to her room. So I kissed Patricia and told her it is going to be all right and I would be here when she gets out, waiting.

While that was happening, I went to get something to eat and go outside to get some fresh air and to talk to Jesus. Thank God I have Jesus to talk to and to help give me strength. To help the doctors and nurses while they worked with Patricia and that this biopsy would come back negative on cancer being in the bone.

The time may have been around 10 PM when they brought Patricia back up to her hospital room. God love her. Patricia was ready to eat, but she would have to wait for the all clear from the nurse. I think it was around midnight. The all clear and plus the anesthesia was wearing off. The cafeteria was already closed. I went out from the hospital and picked up Patricia a hamburger, French fries, and a sprite to drink. Patricia loved it and slept well. For myself, I was living off the hospital cafeteria food and snack bar. Not to mention how expensive that was. It was better for me to stay at the hospital then to drive out and find food and also I was so afraid I would miss something. I even put my cell phone number on the daily board on the wall just in case I was outside and one of the nurses needed to call me. I made sure Patricia's cell phone was charged and by her bed just in case she wanted to call me or the girls or somebody.

When I would step out of the room I would let the nurse's station know that I would be out for a few moments. We would keep the rails up on Patricia's bed and the bed alarm on, just in case,

Patricia tried to get up on her own. Patricia is so independent. I would run home, sometimes from the hospital. It was about 50 minutes away to check on our dog Wally, he is a pretty good dog, he stays outside and he sure has a loud bark, He is a beagle. Especially when somebody was coming up to the house, it would wake you up, that's for sure. I also made sure the lamppost was on every night. If I knew that I was not going to be home for a couple days I would go ahead and leave the lamppost on all night and day, take a shower, get clean clothes, shave, grab some more supplies, and get right back up to the hospital.

The four girls would take turns coming up to the hospital when they could. They all had to work and I understand that. Sometimes I would just need to get out for a little while. We were waiting on the test results to come back on the biopsy. We all were hoping for some good news from that report. My main concern was for Patricia to be comfortable and no worries. I feel that

Patricia did not really understand what was going on with all that was happening with her body and all that medication. Patricia just wanted to go home.

We were going on three weeks of being in the hospital for the second time. We all knew Patricia had been through so much so far. God love her. I asked the nurse if she could find out any news on the biopsy report. She told me it may be another day or two.

The next morning, I got up early and scheduled a service call and then I told Patricia today is a day for rest. I didn't want her to worry about anything, and I was going to run to do a job, go by the house, and check on it. I will be back as soon as possible. She was still pretty weak in her thinking and really needed the rest.

I even went out to tell the nurses' station that I would be gone for four or five hours. I had to go out and do a job and if they would please keep an extra eye on Patricia, she did not sleep well last night. Patricia really needs to rest this morning and please help Patricia order lunch when it became lunch time because it's hard for Patricia to order over the phone. Patricia was resting so well when I left the hospital to go to the job. I just pulled up in the driveway at the house when the phone rang.

It was Patricia. I was really surprised that she was calling me so early. I thought she would have been sleeping. I cannot believe what she was saying to me. Here is what I wrote in my journal. I was hoping it was just a dream.

10/07/2014- Twenty years, five months and three days. The love of my life called me from her hospital bed at 8:40 AM and tells me a doctor had just came in to her room and told her that she was going to die. There is no hope. They were just going to have to control the pain because there is no treatment that can help her or a cure that can save her. The next thing Patricia told me broke my heart. She said I don't want to die. What is that about? I could not believe that the doctor came in and told Patricia something like that with no family member in the room. I told Patricia I bet that was just a dream and stay calm. I would be right back as fast as I can.

After I got off the phone with Patricia I called up to the nurse's station and asked if a doctor had just left visiting in Patricia's room? The nurse looked up on the computer and sure enough, Dr. "O" just left. I told her what he had said to Patricia and she was shocked too. She tells me, "Let me see what he wrote on his notes that were on the computer." It read something like this patient has Stage IV Cancer and it's in the bone. It is inoperable and too late for treatment, just control pain.

Do you see what I say about missing something? I asked the nurse to please send someone into the room and sit with Patricia, that she was by herself and God only knows what she may be thinking. It was ripping out my heart thinking that Patricia was all alone when the doctor tells her she was going to die and there`s nothing they can do about it. I was thinking that, if it wasn't for Patricia being so tired and not thinking real clearly, I don't think she fully understood what was said. Thank God!

On the way back to the hospital I called the oldest daughter and told her what had just happened. I told her what was said to Patricia in the hospital room where she was all alone and how I asked the nurses to please keep a good eye on her. They knew I was going to be out for a while and that she needed to rest.

Melinda was so shocked to hear that. She said that she was going to leave work and come right up to the hospital to be with Patricia. She would call the other three girls and let them know. I feel that when the doctor stepped into the room and seeing there was no family member in the room, he should have gone to the nurse's station to ask if he could have us all together to give the test results. It would have been good protocol to do so. That is not news you would want to give someone that is sick and weak. Not to mention Patricia is having trouble with her thinking. I feel that it would have been better to have a loved one with you to hold your hand and comfort you in a moment like that.

www.EricRoberts-Author.com

I will say again, "It has a lot to do with that word communication!"

Patient, doctors, nurses, aides, lab technicians, loved ones, especially their partners, or their other half needs to be able to communicate. I got to thinking how other patients would have taken news like that and then the doctor just leaves the room. I guess it would depend on their mental state at the time. News like that may have sent someone right out the window. Pardon the pun. I know Patricia was not understanding clearly at the time but I sure wish I had been there when she got the devastating news. God love her! I started praying to the Lord that he send the Holy Spirit and Angels to be with her and help comfort her. I know that Patricia was not really all alone. She had Jesus.

I got back to Patricia's Hospital room as fast as I could. I was glad to see she was resting. I stepped out into the hallway to speak with the head nurse that was on duty at the time and asked if she would please give me the phone number to the Hospital Director. I felt it was time to talk to someone that could make a difference about the communication that really needs to be addressed. I put it in my pocket and got right back in the room to be with Patricia.

Patricia was glad to see all the girls were coming in to be with her. We all were trying so hard to stay positive, especially in front of Patricia and just let her know we all are here and no bad news was going to rob our peace and hope. There were some good things starting to happen. Like the radiation was starting to relieve the pain in Patricia's leg from the tumor pushing on the sciatic nerve and her appetite was coming back. I was so glad to see her eating better. I know Patricia loves to eat. We just kept up the positive reinforcement and tried to stay focused on getting stronger and not give up the fight.

I could see it in Patricia's eyes. She was really leaning towards me to be her helper, we are not giving up and it is in

God's hands. I feel that helps comfort her. I know the love we shared together. We both drew off of each other. I would tell Patricia every day, "I am your Earth Angel!" The whole time we were in the hospital, Patricia was more comfortable when I was changing her sheets to help keep things clean. I even changed the bandages on her back. I would tell her, "Don't you worry about it. That's what true love does." I would say, "You would do the same for me," and she would say, "You know you got that right." That is just the kind of person I am. I guess I got it from my Mama, and believe me, I did not mind at all helping Patricia. I would not have it any other way. Some days were hard, some were easy. Some were sad, some were funny, but we both were in it together and it is in God's hands. We are going to focus on winning.

We talked to the Doctors to see what our next options were. They were talking about sending Hospice in to talk with us. While we were waiting to hear back from Hospice, I got an appointment to speak with the Director of the Hospital. I am usually not so outspoken but I felt I needed to let the hospital know what I was observing. Some big things to some little ones, but it all made a difference. The way I was looking at it was from someone on the outside of the medical industry giving some constructive criticism. I am not mad or wanting anyone to be in trouble, but like a learning moment.

When I got to go in to speak with the Hospital Director I took my notes and went over them with the Director. I told the Director right off I was just there trying to help, and that I was there to be the voice of Patricia about her experience and mine. There is trouble with communication between loved ones, patients, doctors, lab technicians, nurses, specialists, or anyone else that may have to do with the patient's healthcare and the whole experience. I told her that I was just a plumber and not a very smart man but there was thing's I was seeing and hearing that I thought she would be interested in knowing about. I started by reading to the Director my notes and I am going to write them into this story. I am titling it, "From the start Communication."

Nurses working 7 to 7+ hours are pretty tired at the end of their shifts. The hospital not sharing information between the family and the spouse who brought the patient in for care. In the ICU, there was blood on pillow for over three hours. ICU nurse telling patient to keep quiet, or spouse will have to leave and that you will be by yourself. Not good! Ask for help, then over 20 minutes later or sometimes not even coming back. Leaving a clear, open plastic bag of patient's IV, blood transfusion bag in patients sink with toothbrush and personal items on back of sink over two hours. How they sent the wrong medical chart down to biopsy with the wrong name. Caseworker turned in Patricia's case three weeks late to Medicaid. She said she forgot to get it in, causing more delay. No demonstration on how to take care of the nephrostomy tubing and dressing, or how and when to flush tubing. Not enough physical therapy for the patient.

They need more communication between staff on mental state of patient. What needs and concerns are met and how we had waited, and waited, and waited for a procedure. Need to let the patient and family members know some kind of time frame to help calm the patient. Let spouse or family member stay with the patient who knows them best. Listen to what they are saying and make footnotes on the medical charts especially on their mental health or mental strength and weaknesses. For example, if they are having trouble with making clear decisions on their own with the patient's strengths and weaknesses, make sure that all gets communicated thru the whole process and stays with the notes provided.

If there is going to be a possibility for an infection from the patient's condition, they should have a prescription of antibiotics to take home with them to have on standby and how to watch out for the signs of infection. I feel that one big dose of radiation three weeks ago when we were in the hospital the first time, would have helped with three weeks of unnecessary pain and suffering. They need more demonstration on how to care for the patient when you get them home.

I feel that the staff could have done a better job with more positive talk with the patient. They need to smile more, check on the bedding sheets, pillowcases, and the gowns. Don't just ask the patient if they need changing. Most patients say it's OK, but just maybe they're too embarrassed to tell the truth.

They need to communicate the strengths and mental state of the Patient between Care Technicians to the next Care Technicians of the Patient. Like if the Patient is, weak and has trouble with standing and walking, or maybe having trouble with remembering. If needed make sure they get a "FALL RISK" band, on their arm and a yellow hospital gown on. Which, that is recommended, to be put on the patient as soon as it is found out they are a "FALL RISK."

Why am I mentioning this? After seven days from being in the hospital, the head nurse finally caught Patricia was not wearing one, and had ordered one right away for Patricia. I was also wondering what protocol there is after the patient has been lying in the bed for a week and if there should be more work with exercising, sitting up, rolling over side to side or something, so they are not just laying on their back for over a week.

I might have a little invention for when they come in to take a stool sample. I was noticing there was just a Popsicle Stick and when you try to pick up diarrhea with the Popsicle Stick, it is really difficult. I was thinking maybe having a stool spoon that is made out of wood. Like a little spoon that you get with the little ice cream dippers. Especially when you have diarrhea, it's really hard to pick up diarrhea with a Popsicle Stick. Believe me I tried it a couple times. It's just an idea. I mentioned to the Director again that I am just a concerned Plumber and was just trying to help.

I told her of another idea that I had that might help when a new patient comes in to the emergency room. I told the Director it would be of great help if there was a two-person team that could come speak with the patient and the spouse or whoever brings the patient in for care. Separate from the Doctors and Nurses, maybe two women or men or a mix depending on the Patient's gender to take notes to keep with the Medical Chart. A cheerful experience for the Patient! Ask questions like what do you like to eat or drink? What are your hobbies? Do you like sleeping with the lights on or off? Do you sleep on your back or on your side? Who would they like to speak for them on their behalf to Doctors or Nurses? Who will speak with Spouse or Guardians? Maybe just get to know a little more about their mental health. Ask a few questions and probably many more questions that could be asked, just get to know the Patient better. It helps so much with their care and mental health just to listen and communicate.

I also let her know back on Tuesday, 11/08/2014, I had to leave the hospital to do a service call. My oldest daughter was going to come and set with Patricia at 2 PM. I asked the Care Technician and Patricia's Nurse if they would please change Patricia's gown and bedding, it was getting kind of soiled. I left at 1 PM and came back to the hospital about 4 PM. Our daughter pointed out to me that the bedding was soiled. I checked. It was! I told her that I had asked them to please change it all just before I left. Melinda said she would go out to the Nurse's Station and see what happened with that request. Melinda came back into the room and told me that the Nurses came in three different times and asked Patricia if she needed changing and she told them no, she was okay and they just left the room.

I was thinking what is all that about? I told all of them, the Technician and the Nurses that Patricia is having trouble with her thinking, plus all the drugs she is taking. They know she needs help. See there, its communication again. Believe me I did my best to pass that information on from Care Person to Care Person! It just gets lost somewhere. That is why it should be in the notes with their medical chart and better communicated with all involved.

I also told the Director of how they kept coming into Patricia's room to give her stool softener and somehow they just didn`t get that Patricia has diarrhea already and if I was not there they would had just given it to Patricia. That happened five or six times. I had just spoken with the Medical Doctor's Team that was working with Patricia just earlier in the morning about her medication, about her pain level, and how the radiation was working to help with the pain and how I was thinking that the morphine may be too much and maybe if possible let's hold off on the morphine for now, just go with the hydrocodone for the pain. I explained how the morphine was making Patricia so loopy. Plus, it was interfering with Patricia's appetite. How the Doctors agreed with me and thanked me for being the "Voice" for Patricia and they told me Patricia is blessed that I could be here for her.

Well it happens later that afternoon, the Nurse came in to give Patricia her meds and sure enough they were going to give her morphine and stool softener again. I explained to the Nurse how I had spoken with the Doctors earlier and that we were just going to go with the hydrocortisone for now. She called down to the Doctor in charge of Patricia's medical case on the phone and they apologized and said they just have not put it in the computer yet! "Communication," I am so glad I could be there for Patricia. I just do not know if Patricia would have been thinking clearly enough to let them know if she needed certain medications or not.

I also told the Director of the Hospital about how the Doctor that took Patricia's "Biopsy of the Bone," came into her room with no family members there while Patricia was all by herself weak and confused. He told Patricia that there was nothing they could do for her and there is no treatment to cure her. She was just going to die and that they were just going to control her pain. He suggested Patricia going on Hospice. Even the Director was shocked to hear it was handled that way and told me that they would talk with the Doctor. I thanked the Director for her time and said I hope this was a positive meeting. I just wanted to help for the next Patient that comes into the hospital for treatment.

I feel that the Ebola crisis could not have been because of equipment failure, but just maybe because of long shifts and communication breakdown. Then the Director thanked me again and was so glad I brought these concerns to their attention.

When I got back to Patricia's Hospital Room, all the girls were there. They told me that the Hospice Counselor would be in shortly to talk with us about

Patricia going on hospice and they will be sending Patricia home soon. Patricia sure was glad to hear she would be going home soon. I can't blame her. From the first time we were here in the Hospital to now, going on six weeks. That is a lot of "Hospital Time." We were keeping on top of this disease and doing all we could to keep up the good fight, we would tell each other we are doing well. We will do our part and the Doctors will do their part. God is doing his and that's all we could ask for.

Hospice came in and introduced themselves to Patricia, then two of the girls and I went out and sat in the waiting area in the hall way. We filled out paperwork on Hospice and then the Counselor explained how Hospice works and what to expect. They would help with supplies and set up a hospital bed at the house, furnish shower chairs, and any other needs. They were going to help with Patricia's medication that Patricia would be taking each day and a registered nurse would be there to help with pain control.

I asked about payment and how we had no Insurance. I explained how we had a Hospital Social Worker working on getting Patricia on Medicaid. I think it is called Social Security Insurance. The Counselor explained, by Patricia going on Hospice that would speed up the process a little bit more. They would be working close with the Hospital Social Worker to get it moving along and for us not to worry. The paper was drawn out that I would be the one signing the papers and when it came to signing the do not resuscitate order. All the girls were fine with me signing that order. I understand how they felt. I did not mind either. I know Patricia would have done the same for me. This was one of the hardest things I have ever done. It felt that signing up on Hospice was us giving up the fight, but at this time we had no other options.

The Hospital had done all they can do and all they could do was send Patricia home. It was good that it was with hospice because Patricia would be getting a Registered Nurse to come to the house two times a week to keep up with her health condition. That is better than just not doing anything at all. I spoke with the girls before we went back into the Hospital Room and told them do not worry. Their mother would be taken very good care of and that I was going to do everything I could to make sure their mother was getting all that she needs. She was going to be as comfortable as possible. All the girls thanked me and told me they know that I was going to be the best person to take care of their mother. I also know that Patricia is so blessed to have four wonderful daughters. I thank God every day for all four of them. I know that this has been so hard on them seeing their mother like this. It was just so sudden. God love them.

The hospital was going to release Patricia the next morning. It was going to be 01/21/2015, on a Wednesday. The youngest daughter said she would stay with their mother so I could go to the house and get it ready for the Hospice to bring out the bed and supplies the next morning.   That evening I told Patricia I was going to the house tonight to get it cleaned up and all ready for her to come home tomorrow.   That made Patricia so happy, she did not mind me being gone all night. I think she was just happy to be going home. I just got to say at this point, I know God was with us. I never would have thought I would see and witness a person like Patricia with the strength she had to be so calm and hopeful.   I was seeing in Patricia the strong will that she has and I know I am in God's hands too. I know that Jesus gives me my strength and peace that I have and the positive attitude to pass it on to everybody around me. Anytime someone would ask me how I am doing, I would always say, "Fantastic," every day at any time. It helped so much that I had a mother that raised me up in Sunday School and Church. I get it now!

Since the last two weeks we were in the Hospital, Patricia had Angels visit a couple of times. She would wake up and tell me of someone that she had visited with. One day Patricia was lying in the bed and she was talking to her sister Kathy that had passed away three years earlier and she asked me, "Do you not see her? She is right there," pointing at the corner of the Hospital Room. Another time, Patricia was talking to her Father that passed away about 10 years earlier. Patricia told me that he was sitting right there on the bed one morning. I know I believe in Angels and it could have been possible.

I am writing this book for the dignity and the desire to share it with someone in the hopes it may help them in their journeys. One more thing, I would like to mention what happened in the last week we were at the hospital.

One morning when we woke up, I noticed a necklace. It was a beaded necklace that her older daughter Kellie had given Patricia the night before, just hanging there, like it was on a wire. It did not hit the floor. I was thinking no way, that's got to be a miracle, you would have had to see it to believe it. I think the Angels kept it from hitting the floor and that is all I will say about that. I just know there was something or someone in that room, giving her Peace. God love her!

Later that evening I made sure Patricia's cell phone was charged all the way and by her bed. That way she could reach it if she would like to call me later. I gave Patricia a big hug and kiss and told her I'll see you later. I want to go on to the house and get it ready for tomorrow so we can get you home. Patricia was so happy and gave me a big smile. I was so relieved knowing Kristie was going to stay the night with her mother, so she would not be alone. I know Patricia was getting anxious.

It was about 10 o'clock that evening when I got to the house. I just wanted everything to go as smooth as possible so Patricia would be comfortable as possible and for her no worries at all. We both like easy. That is just the way we roll. "We got this," she would say. I felt that Patricia would be most comfortable in our bedroom, so I took down our big bed and put it in the extra room. I made room for some shelves to keep supplies on like sheets, gloves, pads, towels, rags, and medical supplies, just to keep everything handy. Again, we like easy!

I hung a big sign in the bedroom on the wall that said, "I can do all things through Christ who strengthens me." I wanted her bed facing a certain way, so Patricia could look out on the beautiful yard, the lamppost, and she can see her pickup truck in the driveway. It is a little silver Dodge Dakota pickup, the truck Patricia always wanted. I am hoping for anything to give her encouragement to never give up hope in beating this and always thinking to drive on and maintain. Keep God First! God love her! I tried to keep as much of the furniture in place to help Patricia feel right at home.

Patricia loves this place so much, the house, the yard and the smells. Just what the doctor ordered! I went out and bought new sheets, extra pillows, and towels. I even bought a wheelchair, shower chair, and a potty chair, the kind you can set over the toilet if you wanted to and it has arms on each side.

It was about 4 o'clock in the morning when I felt I had everything ready and everything was in place. That is when I hit my knees and open myself up to God thanking him for bringing Patricia this far and giving me the strength and the ability to stay hopeful. I could feel the presence of the Holy Spirit as I went around the house, pleading the Blood of Jesus over everything. I know the Lord does work in mysterious ways and God has a purpose for me to be here at this time. I know it brought the girls and me closer together. I know that I pleaded the Blood over their lives every day just like my mother had done for me. I know the importance to have God in your life and the Holy Spirit to help guide you and comfort you.

The next morning Kristie called me around 8:30 to let me know that they would be releasing Patricia from the hospital around 1 o'clock. The Hospice Supply Truck showed up around 10:30

that morning to set up the bed in the bedroom and air up the mattress. All I could think about was how I bet Patricia is really getting excited about coming home today. The Hospital was going to give Patricia a ride home in the Ambulance, so she would not have to set up all the way home. That is a good thing.

I was sitting out on the front porch when the Ambulance turned into the driveway. I was wondering what was going through Patricia's mind when she knew she was coming down the driveway. I bet Patricia had a big smile on her face. God love her. I know she has been through so much in just the last four weeks. I am so happy to see Patricia home, my best friend and the love of my life. I was as ready as I could be to help in any way knowing I got Jesus to help me and give me knowledge and strength, and don't forget the hope. "HOPE!" I just had to say it again. It feels good to say it.

The paramedics brought Patricia home

The Paramedics brought Patricia into the house on one of those big gurneys on wheels, but it would not go around the corner of the hallway. I told the Paramedics, "Let's just put Patricia on the couch, she should be fine. We can go back to the bed later." Then one Paramedic grabbed one end of the sheet, the other Paramedic grabbed the other end of the sheet and picked Patricia up off the gurney and whisked her onto the couch. It was so funny we all started laughing. Patricia clapped her hands and said, "Let's do it again! Let's do it again!" She is so funny!

Patricia was so happy to be back at home. Patricia said there's my TV, there's my Coffee Table, there's my Hutch, and that's my Coffee Maker. I guess there is no place like Home. It was good to see that her spirits were high. Shoot, I was happy to be back at home myself. Patricia, me, and the dog Wally, that's wonderful! It was so good to see Patricia's mind so sharp and not much pain.

One of the first things Patricia asked me is when do these tubes come out of her back. Patricia hated those nephrostomy tubes that went into her kidneys, but that is the only way she could pass her urine into that bag. I told her we are going to stay on top of that and do all we could do to get them out of her kidneys. Her kidneys were working pretty well, it's just that tumor had been pressing on her bladder and causing them not to work right. Even though, the Radiologist Doctor had told us that the radiation should shrink the tumor and help with the pain in her legs from pressing on the sciatic nerve. Oh, and let's not forget about the diarrhea, lots of diarrhea from the radiation it was to be expected. Although I do believe that the radiation was working.

I know one thing I am so glad we went back to the hospital when we did or it could have been a lot worse. I still feel the hospital could have done more the first time we went back in September when they found out that she had a tumor in her belly. We still have follow-up appointments that Patricia would have to follow up on and I was going to make sure to get Patricia to each one. I wanted to ask all the right questions when we go in for those appointments. I wanted to see what we would have to do to get these nephrostomy tubes taken out of Patricia as soon as possible.

While Kristie is here I thought I would run to the grocery store and pick up a few things. I asked Patricia what I could get her from the store she said, "Cake, lots of cake." Well that's what it's going to be. I came home with five cake mixes, chocolate cake, lemon cake, yellow cake, and white cake. Cake, lots of cake! That first day home I made a chocolate cake. Patricia ate three big slices right off the bat and had a big glass of ice cold milk. What a smile! God I love this woman so much. It was so good to see her eating good.

Patricia has some favorite shows she likes to watch on TV and she tried to catch each one of them each chance she got. Patricia would just laugh and laugh at all the characters, especially that Sheldon. She thought he was so funny. Here is some of Patricia's other likes. Ellen, The Price is Right, How I met your Mother, Mike and Molly, Two Broke Girls, The Talk, The View, and Kellie and Michael in the mornings. She likes Supernatural, The Green Arrow, and she had her favorite soap operas she would watch. We sure enjoy each other's company.

We would talk about our lives when we were growing up. She was born in Ohio and moved to Texas when she was around nine or 10 years old. She grew up going to Sunday School and her dad played in the band with her and her three sisters singing in the choir. It was nice to hear that we both grew up with almost the same upbringings and how we had great parents that knew the importance of knowing God.

God sent his Son to be our helper and Savior and how he died on the cross for our salvation, grace and forgiveness. I will always know that even though Patricia, for a while had strayed from God for a time in her life, The Holy Spirit and I know God was working his plan in Patricia's life, her body, and her soul. I could see in Patricia that she is growing a closer walk with Jesus. The Peace, Joy, and the Hope she was experiencing while all this was happening in her life. It is a deep divine experience for both of us.

The friendship and true love we share is a blessing from above and it's in God's hands. We would talk about how it was meant for us to meet and how no matter what was going on that our motto was going to be never giving up. That first night from the hospital Patricia slept on the couch. I slept on the floor beside her and I was happy to be home too!

Let me tell you that stay at the hospital stretched me pretty thin. I am not complaining, but we both could have gone without all that, if you know what I mean?   I did learn the ropes at the hospital, like learning where the cafeteria is, how to find the parking lot, and where the vending machines were in that big hospital.   Let me tell you two months of that will wear you out.   Thank God the girls were there to help out when they could.   I know they all were still young and have lives, jobs, and responsibilities they had to take care of.   I know it was all a burdening on them too. God love them. Let me mention the food prices at the hospital are expensive and that's just for me.   Patricia got to eat off the hospital menu.

The next day Hospice came out to the house.   We met the Registered Nurse, the Chaplain, and the Bath Lady.   Patricia and I would just call her Ms. Rita.   Ms. Rita and Patricia hit it off right away and you will see they became best friends! Then the Nurse checked Patricia all out for her vital signs, her temperature, and her blood pressure.   Everything looked real good.   Even her urine got the all clear. Ms. Rita said she would come back next week to see if Patricia needed some help bathing. She is a very nice lady and she's funny.

Now to get to the Chaplain, the Chaplain visited with us. I found out you had to call him Chaplain, not a Pastor or any other name. It just had to be Chaplain.

It's not like the time back when we grew up. I never thought I would see the day when the Preacher would come to visit with a tablet computer instead of having a Holy Bible. With no interference Christian Fellowship meeting, you would have to go through a checklist of questions on a computer and have to answer each question before you can move on to the next one. You have to be careful not to discriminate on how you answer the question. What's that about? It was a learning moment.

I explained to the Chaplain there was a lot of this I was seeing in the Hospital. That's a great tool but something is getting lost along the way from this technology and there should be more personal relationship with the Patient, close Family, and Spouses or just the person that knows the Patient best. More could be done to combine the two together. I mentioned to the Chaplain that I had spoken with the Director of the Hospital on them just focusing on the diagnosis, keeping up with the medication, and vital signs logged in on the computer.

Something needs to be set up with a separate Psychology Team to meet with Patients and Spouse or whoever comes in with the Patient. To keep foot notes on the mental state of the Patient and to keep it in their charts along with the medical records, it helps with their healthcare. It also could help from somebody falling down and getting seriously hurt.

I feel there will never be a computer of any kind of technology that would ever take the place for one on one human connection to overcome humanity and express the love and compassion we need for one another. We need this with one another and I feel it is only going to get worse over the next few years as our hospitals start getting more overworked. I can just hope that maybe someone that reads this book can see the importance of working closer with the patient's mental state and physical weaknesses.

Sometimes Patients need to rely on someone because of some reasons like being unconscious, sedated, or maybe in a coma or just from all the different medications. All I am trying to relay is try to find out something about the Patient they are treating. They should pass this information on between Caregiver to Caregiver, Nurse to Nurse, Technician to Technician, Specialist to Specialist, and Doctor to Doctor. There is something here that it is being missed and needs to be addressed quickly! I also want to mention that some things that need to be communicated can be lost between shifts, too. Doctors and Nurses need to be more "SENSTIVE" towards the "MENTAL STRENTH" of all Patients.

I want to mention of an idea I have, it could put more Psychologists to work. Put a two-person team together that could meet with each Patient that comes into the Emergency Room and visit with the Patient. It could be 2 males 2 females or you can mix depending on the gender of the Patient and maybe their age, or nationality. You could call this Psychology Team the "M.H.S.E.T.," that stands for "Mental Health State Evaluation Team." It would be better for a two-person team. One may catch something that the other did not. I just wanted to put that in there.

My Wife would have done the same for me. God bless her. Let me tell you if you ever have a loved one that has to go into the Hospital and they are not thinking clearly for whatever reason, stay with them, let everyone that is in their care giving know if they are weak, uncomfortable, or have trouble standing, walking, or just needs extra attention! For now, it is GETTING LOST and that is all I will say about that for now.

Now that I talked the Chaplain's leg off, we had a nice little prayer with Patricia. The Hospice Chaplain was very understanding and a very nice person. The Chaplain gave us his phone number in case we ever felt like we needed prayer. We were free to call it any time day or night. All of the Hospice Staff was helpful to us and all of them showed a positive attitude, which is outstanding.

Teaching myself to be a Healthcare worker

I was teaching myself to be a healthcare worker and even started a daily journal at home about the Hospital.

Home Sweet Home, 11-12-15 Patricia Fraley at 4:30 AM, Tylenol for pain in right side of her neck may be due from a new bed and new pillow. Still having diarrhea from radiation treatment! 7:30 AM-1 slow-release iron, 2 sodium bicarbonates, one 500 mg vitamin C, 1 Centrum vitamin supplement. 8:30 AM - For breakfast 4 bites of eggs and had a piece of toast with butter, 2 cups of vitamin D milk. 1:00 PM- for lunch a half of peanut butter and jelly sandwich and a half a cup of milk. Meds - two sodium bicarbonates, 5 PM 1 bag of 1 ounce Keebler Chips Deluxe mini cookies, so good! Oh boy! Still has diarrhea. 6:45 PM- ate half of a homemade cheeseburger and had 1 cup of vitamin D milk. 7:30 PM- move from couch to bed 7:45 PM- I would list the five medications she was taking. Then I would take Patricia's blood pressure, her pulse, and her temperature and log it down 8:00 PM- big slice of yellow cake with chocolate frosting, with 1 cup of vitamin D milk, oh so good! No pain, yes. Good night my love. 9:45 PM- sleeping well.

The next day I would start a new log. I felt that keeping a daily log helps for things to go easier and just in case the Registered Nurse or the Doctors need to keep up with Patricia`s progress at home. While we were in the Hospital, I was learning each day taking it all in. Each time the Medical Staff would come into Patricia's hospital room I asked questions. I was eager to learn so I could be the best I can be to help Patricia beat this sickness. The love that Patricia and I shared together is a love of unconditional Peace and Hope. The love that we share is working in our spirits. It is RARE! We share a wonderful friendship and we are living each day as if this was going to be the day for healing.

Each morning Patricia and I would wake up around 4:30 AM, sometimes 5 AM. Like clockwork, one of us would have gotten the coffee pot ready for the next morning all you would have to do is push the button. We like easy. Patricia was working more with getting around with the Walker. I feel that she could have gotten around without it. I think it was more of a security blanket. God love her. Plus, she could hang her nephrostomy tube bag on it and use both hands on the Walker and that's okay, its progress. Seeing her eating better and all that medication was wearing off from the hospital stay.

By 11/19/2014, she was walking back and forth from the living room to the hospital bed that was set up in our bedroom. Sometimes Patricia and I would have our coffee in the bedroom where she could set up in the bed and look out the bedroom window. We would watch the sun come up. I had a chair where I could sit beside the bed so we would watch the early news, enjoy our coffee and each other's company. Thank goodness the diarrhea was going away, she was almost back to normal. This was unimaginable what Patricia and I went through with that hurdle in the hospital, up till now. Need I say more? Let's move on.

Patricia and I did not talk about any cancer. I guess we did not want to look at her situation as battling cancer but to focus more on beating the tubes in her back. She hated having them there. If they could just come out, she could get around better and that would help with her healing so much more. Patricia called it her ball and chain. We would stay as positive as we could. We knew she had an appointment coming up soon to see the oncologist. Then we could talk to him about seeing what we can do to get them removed since her kidneys are working fine.

The tumor has shrunk pretty well. Even her urine was all the right shades. Patricia told me that she was so blessed that I was here to help her keep up with all she was going through. She would say often, "Thank you my Love, you are my Soul Mate." I would tell Patricia, "I love you, too. You are my love, my friend." We both know we are soul mates and I would tell Patricia I was her earth Angel.

We were going on 12 days being back from the Hospital for the second time. The Hospice Registered Nurse was pretty amazed how Patricia was doing. Patricia was doing a very good job of taking her medication every day, right on time. She only had to take the pain pills if she really needed to for her leg pain and that was getting lower, too. That was great!

I would help Patricia sit up to take a shower. Patricia is pretty good walking into the bathroom with her walker but I would make sure to help her get in and out of the shower chair. I made sure everything was right in reach. I would help her to dry off and get dressed. After a shower, I would change out Patricia's bandages on her back where her tubing went into her kidneys. We always made sure they stayed covered up and clean. I know it is uncomfortable for her, but we were going to make sure nothing was going wrong.

When Ms. Rita the Hospice Bath Lady would come out to visit Patricia for her bath, we let her know that Patricia was more comfortable if I would bath her. Miss Rita said she did not mind and understood. If at any time Patricia needed her, just let her know and she would be right there, we could call her anytime.

Miss Rita is a very nice lady. Patricia really enjoyed her company. When she would come out they would laugh and joke together. They would talk about old times when they were children and how they were growing up. She was a real blessing for Patricia. They even talked about Jesus sometimes. If I was at home, I would just go on the porch and give them a little bit of lady time. Usually after about 30 minutes, Miss. Rita would leave and Patricia would say she sure enjoyed Miss. Rita's company. Patricia just thought she was a sweet lady.

I was doing the best I could to make sure all the appointments were being kept up. In the living room, over the couch, we kept one of them big white boards that we can write on. It started out with each day of the week and the date under that we would write in schedules of appointments we had with different specialists. We made a list of all Patricia's medications and the times she was supposed to take them. At the bottom, I would write in big letters, "FALL RISK," so that if any one came in, they could see it. Also, Patricia could see it right there when she was on the couch and it helps Patricia to keep up with what was going on. We like easy.

Patricia was starting to get strong enough that I could go out and run a few service calls so we could keep the lights on. Since Patricia did not have a free hand to carry anything when she uses her walker, I hung a bag on her walker. Patricia could carry her cell phone, her bottle water or maybe a book from room to room in it. After we would have our coffee and breakfast, I would lay out

Patricia's toothbrush, water, and something for her to rinse in. We had our own little system set up. Then she would take her morning vitamins and medication. Both of us have been taking our morning vitamins religiously for a long time.

I would make Patricia something for lunch, a snack cake, and something to drink on the coffee table in front of the couch if that is where Patricia was going to be for the day. I would always leave Patricia a note on the coffee table to drink lots of water and exercise. I would put out her medication that she was supposed to take at certain time of the day, put a circle around the medication with an arrow towards it and what time to take it. That was our little system and it was working. I would give her the biggest hug and kiss and tell her to have a wonderful day and I will be back as soon as I can. Patricia would always say, "Be careful," and I would say, "Always." We always ended our phone conversation that way. We have been doing that for years.

Thanksgiving was coming up and pumpkin pie was all Patricia could think about with Cool Whip on top. All the girls wanted to have Thanksgiving at our house and said they would take care of it all. Patricia was getting pretty excited about all the food. Her appetite was really doing well. I loved seeing her eat so well.

Kristie our youngest daughter came over three days before Thanksgiving. She wanted to color her mama's hair. Patricia was so excited about that, they had fun. Patricia got her hair colored right there in the hospice bed. I enjoyed watching them.

It was a wonderful Thanksgiving. All that food! Kristie catered the turkey and dressing and all the other girls brought dishes of food. There was so much food, Patricia ate well and a she had a wonderful time! We all did. I knew what was going on in the back of all of our minds, this might be the last Thanksgiving we would get to share with Patricia. This was going to be the finest and best we ever had. That was for sure!

We all kept a good attitude and made sure we all stayed positive. God love her. We all encouraged Patricia and we all let Patricia know we loved her so much. None of us wanted her in any pain and so far it was keeping under control. Thank God!

Patricia's appointment was coming up soon with the doctor that put in the nephrostomy tubing in to her kidneys, they were due to be replaced and Patricia was ready to get it done. This was more of a follow-up procedure. As long as Patricia is on Hospice she is not allowed to take any kind of treatments. Hospice does not pay for that. They would cover the follow-up appointments only. Patricia would have to go under anesthesia to have the procedure done on her. Patricia would not be able to eat or drink anything the day before her appointment. Patricia would say, "I got this." I sure do admire her passion and desire to get through this. We both would often say, "THIS TOO SHALL PASS."

Hospice is doing such a fine job, anything Patricia needed we just had to ask them. If Patricia was running low on her medication, the Hospice Registered Nurse made sure it was ordered early enough that it would be at the house the same day or the next. It was so much of a blessing that Hospice is here. If I ever needed prayer, I could call the Chaplain and he would pray for me right over the phone.

Sometimes the Chaplain would come out to the house to pray with us both, Patricia and I. Patricia enjoyed talking with the Chaplain about the Lord. I could see that Patricia was getting closer to God. **He was there the whole time.** I know in my heart that Patricia is saved by the grace of God. For whatever reason that this was happening in Patricia's life with this sickness, the Holy Spirit is with her, to comfort her and to be her helper.

I know God is listening to her prayers because one day I was walking through the living room going into the kitchen, when Patricia was laying there on the couch watching her early morning shows.   Patricia muted the TV and pointed up at me and said I prayed for your leg so it would heal. I said you did! I was thinking to myself, with all that Patricia is going through, she is praying for me to heal. God love her.

You see, four days before that I had stepped into a hole at work and twisted my knee, and it was hurting so much I had to put ice packs on it as much as I could to help keep the swelling down. It was pretty hard for me to walk. Then just two hours after that, Patricia had prayed for my knee to stop hurting. It was a miracle! I know this because **PATRICIA SAID A PRAYER FOR ME**. You know that for the last 19 years that Patricia and I have been together. I think that's the first time she has ever told me she said a prayer for me. God love her. I thank God every day for Patricia and put my trust in him. That helps give me, my peace that surpasses all understanding and her praying for me confirms that we are meant to be together at this time in our lives to be each other's helper.

The day before Patricia was supposed to go in for her procedure. Patricia was doing a good job not eating anything, but she could drink water. We did have our morning coffee, that's cheating just a little bit, I Know! We had to have our coffee. We were addicted and couldn't help ourselves. That evening, I was so proud of Patricia. I laid out some clothes in the bathroom and asked if I could help her. Patricia said no, "I got this," so she went in there and got into the shower chair by herself, then got out of the shower, and got dressed. She came back to the couch all by herself using the walker to hang her bag on. I was so happy to see the strength that Patricia had, she is so amazing. It was good Patricia had an appointment coming up. Plus, we were going to be able to talk to the Doctor about what we were going to have to do to get those tubes removed. I know she was ready.

The day of Patricia's Appointment

On the day of Patricia's appointment I mentioned to the Doctor that Patricia really did not like those nephrostomy tubes too much and what can we do to get them out. He said after he does the procedure to replaces the tubes, he would shoot die into her tubing. That is called an x-ray dye. He can see if Patricia was going to be able to pass urine on her own without the tubes and he would let me know after that.

Patricia and I really liked this Urologist Doctor. He always had been very straightforward with us, honest, and always had concerns for our needs. The Doctor was very good to explain to Patricia and me how the procedure was going to work. He told us what he was going to do and that under the anesthesia that she would not feel anything. Throughout all of this, the Doctors, the Nurses, and Staff did a very outstanding job. I thanked the Doctor for being so informative to Patricia and me. Then the Dr. told us it would be about two hours and I can wait out in the lobby. I told Patricia, "I love you and I will be right here when you get out, and be waiting!" I went out and waited in the lobby. It was going to be about two hours. Because of the anesthesia, Patricia would need an hour to come out of it.

After the procedure they let me go back to sit with Patricia while she was coming out of her anesthesia. The Doctor came in to talk with us and said everything went just fine. He ran the x-ray dye and told us it looked like urine would still have a little trouble going through. We might have to wait just a little bit longer on getting the tubes removed from her kidneys.

He also explained to us that Patricia had some stents in her bladder and that was holding some things from moving forward. We would have to talk to Dr. Miller. I said "Dr. Miller? I never heard of a Dr. Miller? I did not know anything about stents in Patricia's bladder?" This whole time I made sure Patricia was following up on all her appointments to all the specialists. Everything was being done in the right order and we were doing all that we can do to get her healthier to fight this disease. I know that the doctor that was working with Patricia's nephrostomy tubing in her kidneys was doing all he could do. The Dr. gave me Dr. Miller's phone number and said you need to call Dr. Miller and set an appointment up to talk with him about those stents that Patricia's has in her bladder.

Leaving the clinic, I was still in shock. I was racking my brain trying to remember when Patricia seen a Dr. Miller in the hospital. I was not there that day or I was a sleep. I sure missed that one or I sure would have taken Patricia back for a follow-up to see this Dr. Miller.

On the way back home Patricia and I were still being positive thinking. I know Patricia was looking forward to getting some good news on those tubes coming out soon. I told Patricia when we get home we can call about setting appointment up to see this Dr. Miller and see what needs to be done about those stents that are in your bladder. God love her. We are going to do what we have been doing and that is just keep moving forward. We got this. I admire her strength so much. She is such a blessing.

Just three days later, Patricia was running a hundred and three almost 104 temperatures so I called the Hospice and Registered Nurse to let her know what Patricia's temperature was running. She came right out to the house and took Patricia's temperature and told us it would probably be best that Patricia went back to the Emergency Room at the Dallas Hospital where she was before and call the doctor. Let them know how he just changed out the tubes and there might be an infection and we were on our way. Here we go!

This makes the third time to go back to the hospital. Patricia and I were ready this time we loaded up the wheelchair, packed a bag with some clothes and a tooth brush, all the medications, and all the paperwork we would need to show. It sure helps to make things go smoothly. Then Patricia was ready to go. I went to go out and open the door on the truck and before the time I got back to the house, Patricia had already walked to the front door with her walker. I carried Patricia from there to the truck. It just made it easier. We would have the wheelchair to use when we got to the hospital.

At this point, we felt like we were fighting more than just a tumor and cancer. She was fighting more with the fever and the infections. Patricia wrestling with those tubes while having to carry that bag around on her walker but Patricia is a fighter. She kept up the hope.

When we arrived to the Hospital Emergency Entrance, I got the wheelchair out behind the seat, got Patricia all loaded up, hung her overnight bag that had all we would need in it on to the wheelchair. Then I paid the Valet to park the truck.

We went right to the Emergency Room Reception Desk and checked in. Patricia and I were thinking, "Geez, we've done this before, but we were ready." All the Emergency Health Care Workers were so nice and they all were very respectful towards our needs and concerns.

It wasn't maybe just 15 minutes and we were back in the room waiting to see a Doctor, which was pretty fast. When the Nurses came in to take Patricia's temperature and vital signs, I was sure to point out the yellow wristband to put on Patricia's arm, "FALL RISK," and that she was weak. Patricia's fever was running about 103. It was very concerning. They even took some of Patricia's blood for a blood test. The Doctor came in and talked to us about taking an X-Ray or a CAT scan of Patricia's lower body to see what was causing the infection. I called the girls on cell phone to let them know that I had their mother back up at the hospital and we were having some tests run, something is causing an infection in her body.

Kellie, Patricia's older daughter arrived to the hospital around 8 o'clock am. I told her we were still waiting on test results from her mother's blood test. When Kellie came into the room, Patricia said "Hey, there's my Kellogg's, Momma's little Corn Flake," that is Kellie's nickname from Patricia. I told Kellie I can't believe your mother is going through all this with the tumor and the cancer and here we are back in the Hospital fighting fever and infections. I knew Kellie could see that her Mother has such a strong will, desire, and compassion for life. She has a wonderful attitude, always cheerful, always kind, and courteous to others. Patricia is an amazing lady.

First the X-Ray test results came back, it showed that the stents Patricia had in her bladder were inflamed and causing her high fever. This was most likely what was causing the infection and that it would be a little longer on getting the blood test results back. They were going to move Patricia to her own room.

The Hospital put Patricia over at the Women's Cancer Center wing of the Hospital. It was a really nice room. It had nice wooden floors and a fridge. She even had her own coffee pot right there in the room. It was almost like staying at a fine Hotel. The Medical Staff working over there was so polite and kind to us. They were always asking if there's anything they can do and to let them know, they were there to help.

We were still waiting on test results to come back to see what kind of infection Patricia had in her body. They ended up having to call the Center for Disease Control to analyze what kind of antibiotics they would have to make to get her started on right away. Her temperature would get up to hundred and four. I think that first day Patricia got five different kinds of antibiotics started into an IV. They did this a few times while we were here at the Hospital. They were having a hard time finding Patricia's blood veins to get the IV started. Plus, with all the blood tests since the first time we were in the hospital, up till now, I think they probably stuck Patricia with a needle almost at least 50 times. They were wearing her arms out. I do not think I would have lasted three times.

By this time, we were getting very familiar with how to order food off the Menu and call down to the Cafeteria to let them know what she would like to eat. Patricia almost knew the whole menu by heart. By this time, I guess it has been going on almost 4 months of Hospital time, I feel for anybody that would have to go thru this experience. God love them and their families. I think they must have tried 10 different antibiotics on Patricia trying to get that infection under control. I have never seen anything like it in my life.

On the third day, the Doctor that had put the stents in Patricia's bladder came in to speak with us about what he could do. That was the first time I have ever met Dr. Miller and boy, I have some questions. I pulled out Patricia's paperwork and showed him that nowhere on this paperwork was there ever a follow-up appointment set up to come back to see him about the stents that are in Patricia's bladder. I explained to him how I was keeping up with Patricia's home healthcare, making sure that all of her appointments were being met. That way we could do everything we could to fight this disease and now we find out about the stents.

It seems like just when Patricia is getting stronger and looks like we were winning, something like this comes along to knock Patricia back down again. Also, how we were working close with the Doctor that was working on Patricia's nephrostomy tubes in her back. We were trying to get them out and it looks like this might be holding it up. I was just letting him know that I was not too happy about it. I wanted to know what he is going to do to fix it so we can get Patricia back on her feet again.

Dr. Miller explained to us how he was going to wait three more days until the infection is under control and then he was going to try to take the stents out of Patricia. He explained there were two stents and they would have to come out through her urethra. Then the Doctor explained to us how if he starts the procedure and it looks like too much tissue has grown around the stents, he would not be able to remove them.

I am thinking, oh my God, poor Patricia, she is probably wondering what is going on here. I guess when they had put the stents into Patricia somebody dropped the ball on getting a follow-up appointment set up for her. This is a pretty serious procedure this Doctor is fixing to perform on Patricia. Believe me if I would have known about this earlier, we sure would have been in taking care of it.

I called the Hospice Nurse from the Hospital to keep her updated on Patricia's condition. I explained to the Hospice Nurse about the stents that were left in Patricia's bladder that somebody had forgotten about. She was shocked to hear that. She said she understood about me being so concerned. She has seen

Patricia's paperwork and knew that none of it explained about the stents or a follow-up procedure.

That Saturday, 01/18/2015 Patricia's infection was looking pretty good. It looked like it is getting under control. Dr. Miller set up for Patricia to go in on the 20th and he was going to try to remove the stents early that morning.

Patricia's legs had gotten pretty swollen! I guess from all the IVs. They took Patricia down to do a sonogram on her legs to make sure there were no clots. The results came back all clear. Everybody I asked said they could not explain why her legs were swollen. I had my theory. I think it was from all the IV drips they gave Patricia for the last four days. I counted at least 30. I guess that would make anybody swell up that has been lying in bed for seven days. It all went into Patricia's legs. I am just a plumber but something tells me that is a lot of fluid. It had to be going somewhere. I tried not to worry about that too much. Then sure enough, three days later after they had stopped giving her all those IVs the swelling went back down in Patricia's legs, almost back to normal. God love her.

I know she's going through so much. It is amazing, her strength and will and hopes that Patricia has always shown even up to now through all this. I love this woman so much and she is my inspiration. The night before Patricia's procedure, they told us no eating anything tonight. That sure is tuff on those nights when you do not get to eat. I would go down and find a snack or something, but I feel so bad that Patricia would not get anything to eat. She was quite a good trooper.

www.EricRoberts-Author.com

Hoping and Praying for Good News

Patricia and I was hoping and praying that after the stents come out, maybe then we can start working on getting those tubes out of her kidneys. Patricia would always say they were her "BALL AND CHAIN." We had a good visit with each other that evening and we even had a good prayer together praying that God will keep watching over her. No matter what, we were going to get through this and we prayed for the doctors to do what they had to do.

The next morning, they came to pick Patricia up to take her down to surgery. Believe me I stayed right there beside the gurney while they pushed her down there. I was holding Patricia's hand and encouraging her that it is going to be all right. Then she looked up at me and said, "I got this." God love her strengths!

While we were waiting for them to come and pick up Patricia to take her back for her surgery the Doctor came in and explained to us exactly what he was going to do and assured us again. He was going to try his best to get those stents out. The Doctor told us she would be getting anesthesia and the procedure would take about an hour. Then it would be about another hour for the anesthesia to wear off and I could wait out in the waiting area. They would come get me when they are finished with Patricia.

That's when I went down to the Hospital Chapel and I was praying for almost an hour for the Angels to be there with Patricia while the doctor worked on her. I was praying that this would come out successfully. That would be such a blessing. Lord knew we did not need any more trouble. Patricia has been through so much so far. I was thinking, here we are up at the Hospital again and it was looking like Patricia was having more trouble with complications from other things than what she was diagnosed with. Some of it has to do with that word again, "COMMUNICATION."

Author Eric E. Roberts

Two hours had gone by, and the Doctor came out to the lobby waiting area of the Hospital to speak with me about Patricia's procedure. He explained to me how the procedure went very well. He was able to take the stents out with no problems, and it looks like everything is going to be okay with that. I guess the thing that got me most, is when he tells me, "That's just one less thing you have to worry about." I will not say what I was thinking. It had to do with slapping. For now, I will just keep it to myself. I just know this could have been avoided with better communication.

After three more weeks in the hospital we were ready to head home. Patricia was strong enough that I could push her in the wheelchair to the truck and load up all of her things then off we went. Patricia was so happy to be going home again.   Patricia had a new prescription of antibiotics to take, to add on to all the medication she was taking, if I have not mentioned it yet. Patricia does not like taking medication. I am the same way. Patricia and I just like taking our vitamins and now here she is taking all this medication. At this point in the story about "Patricia's Voice," I can only hope that I can express all that Patricia has been going thru up to this point, it is amazing. We still are keeping a very positive attitude.

After three or four days back home from the hospital, Patricia was back to working out with her little 3 pound weights doing leg exercises, doing anything she could to come back strong. I am so proud of her.

The Hospice Nurse came out to check on Patricia and checked all her vital signs and said they are looking pretty good. She was amazed at what Patricia just went through at the Hospital and Patricia doing as well as she is now. I showed her Patricia's paperwork and nowhere on it mentioned anything about any stents being put in Patricia's bladder.

She told me she knew that it was not my fault because I have been doing such a wonderful job of keeping up with Patricia's care. She can see how much Patricia and I love each other and really care for one another. She told us that Patricia and I were RARE. She has been doing this for 20 years and has never seen a man take as good a care of his wife as I was doing and that made me feel pretty good. It was almost like a compliment. I told her I do this because I know that Patricia would have done the same for me.

Four months later, Medicaid finally kicked in. That made us so happy, thinking maybe now we have more options. Then maybe can get Patricia off Hospice and start treating the cancer with some low dose chemo or something. It was worth a try.

Patricia and I had an appointment set up to see the Radiologist in about two more weeks. We were thinking maybe we can see what he could do with more radiation. So far it has been working pretty well. It was also nice that Medicaid was going to pick up all the hospital bills back from four months ago till now, that is such a relief. Patricia and I both know there was no way we would be able to afford all of those expenses.

It was time to go back for Patricia's follow-up appointment with the radiologist. We were eager to see what he had to say. After we arrived there, I got Patricia loaded into her wheelchair. Patricia was sitting up and looked so strong and eager. We talked to the Radiation Doctor about how the radiation was doing so well and seemed like it had been working just like you said it would.

We asked what we could do now and how we would like to get Patricia off hospice because we have Medicaid now, maybe we can pay for some kind of treatments. He seemed to be pretty amazed at Patricia's progress himself. He explained to us, maybe with some low-dose chemo treatments and maybe another dose of radiation might really be beneficial for Patricia's healing. He told us he would call next door to the Texas Oncology. He knew one of the Doctors over there and would put in a good word for Patricia.

Then he went out into the hallway to make the phone call to next door. Patricia and I could hear what he was saying to the doctor. He was saying that he had a good feeling about this patient and that she was young and she was only 49. He wanted to know if she would mind taking Patricia as one of her clients. It was almost like he was pleading the case for Patricia. That made Patricia and I feel so good. I looked over at Patricia she had a big smile on her face, what he was saying about her, and how he felt she had a pretty good chance. The doctor came back into the room and gave us the phone number of the doctor next door. The Doctor was going to be a woman doctor, after that we left his office.

I wheeled Patricia next door to talk to the nurse's station to make an appointment for Patricia and explain to them how we were on hospice. We now have a Medicaid card and wanted to see what we had to do to get off hospice and set up an appointment to see this lady doctor. The receptionist told us they would call us in the next day or two to let us know about an appointment.

Patricia and I were so excited all the way home we talked about how this is great. Now we got Medicaid, let's get off hospice and see what we can do to speed this healing process up, get some kind of treatment started or something.

As soon as we got back home I called the Hospice Counselor and asked if she would come out to visit with us about signing Patricia off of hospice. The Hospice Counselor was so nice. She was happy to help in any way she was able to. She could see how excited we were of maybe getting something started. All the Hospice Team was rooting for Patricia. The Hospice Counselor got us all signed off of hospice.

Signed off of Hospice

I called back up to the Texas Oncology to see how our appointment was going. That was on a Tuesday and Patricia's appointment was going to be set up for the following Tuesday to see this new Doctor. Patricia and I were glad it was going to be a woman doctor, maybe get some new insights and some fresh eyes to look at her case. I took down the hospice bed and put our queen size bed back up in our room, it was so nice to wake up with Patricia beside me in the morning again. It's been almost 6 months since we have slept together, I held on to Patricia all night long. God I LOVE this woman so much.

The following Tuesday, Patricia and I got loaded up and we were heading to the appointment. The appointment was going to be early like at 8:30 in the morning, so we had to leave about 7 o'clock that morning to have time because we know there was going to be traffic.

We were almost halfway up to the clinic for Patricia's appointment when the secretary called us on the phone. She was explaining how Dr. "O" had spoken with the other Dr. and was wondering why Patricia did not want to go back to see Dr. "O". I explained to her how the radiation doctor had sent Patricia up to see this lady doctor and we did not know that Dr. "O" was working out of that office. The receptionist explained to us that after Dr. W. went over Patricia's case she felt that Patricia would be better served going back to see Dr. "O". I told her I guess it wouldn't matter which doctor we seen, it is just good that Patricia get back in to get some kind of chemo treatments. The receptionist told us please do not come in this morning we will have to call you back with a new appointment to see Dr. "O".

Patricia and I decided to eat and pulled into a donut store. We got us some pig in the blankets, some doughnuts, and headed back to the house. I did not want Patricia to know but in my mind I was thinking that's just great. This is the same doctor that sent Patricia home the first time, and said that she was going to die, because there are no treatments for her. That is kind ironic if you ask me. I explained to Patricia that we are still going to get treatment but just going to see a different doctor.

I feel that Patricia really did not understand that this was the same Dr. "O" that we saw four months ago and all the things that he had told her while she was in the hospital. There was so much going on the last time Patricia was in the hospital, with medication, and with her thinking. Patricia probably would not remember all those things he said to her about there not being any treatment and that she was just going to die. I was looking forward to Patricia seeing a new doctor and her being a woman was even better. Just getting Patricia's foot back in the door at the Texas Oncology and getting off Hospice, it sure was worth a try. I was going to make sure my eyes were wide open when we went back to see this doctor again. I even had a thought that maybe this doctor wanted to keep this case close to his chest. I think you know what I mean?

We made it to the appointment at the Texas Oncology to see Dr. "O" and we got right in. They took Patricia back to a room. I was with Patricia all the way. I wanted to hear what he had to say. Dr. "O" came in the room and said you are looking much better Miss. Patricia. Let's see what we can do to get the nephrostomy tubes out.

Then he asked, "When was the last time Patricia had a radiation treatment?" We explained to him it was about two months ago and how it seemed to be working with the pain. Dr. "O" explained to us he would rather wait three months from after the last RADIATION treatment before he started any kind of treatment for Patricia on chemo and set Patricia up with a new appointment one month from today. That was going to be on April 29, 2015.

He also told us on that appointment that Patricia would be getting a PAP Scan, a new blood test, and then the Dr. wrote Patricia a new prescription for some pain pills and some low dose morphine 30 MG for Patricia to take 1 tablet by mouth every 12 hours. The pain pills are supposed to last for almost a month. Then he left the room.

I do not think the Dr. was in the room for no more than seven minutes. Patricia and I were getting pretty excited knowing we are off of hospice and it looks like we finally are going to get some kind of treatment, but have to wait another month. That's just more DELAY. It's almost 6 months now since we found out Patricia had been diagnosed with a Stage III-B Squamous Cell Cancer of the Cervix. God love her. All the family was so admired of Patricia's strong will, her hope, and her peace. Patricia had such a strong desire to get through this, no matter what.

With Easter coming up, it was going to fall on April 6. Patricia and I figured this year we would just make all 4 of the girls Easter baskets for their whole families. Patricia told me, "If you go get all the baskets and all the goodies to go in them, I will make them up." I said, "Sure Thing." By this time, I had our bed set back up in our room Patricia sure loves that bed. It is a big old queen-size bed. I built a platform beside the bed 6 inches high. It made it easier for Patricia to get up and down onto the bed. The bed is pretty high off the floor when she did walk into the room with her walker. Patricia just had one step up and enough room to walk over to the bed to turn around. Patricia was so thankful. Patricia really enjoyed putting all the Easter baskets together. Patricia sat there on the bed and put all four of them together. I made sure to get plenty of cell phone pictures. God love her.

One week went by from Easter. The clinic called us back and moved Patricia's appointment up for the PAP Scan to the 15th of the month. I would have to take Patricia to the Baylor Hospital in downtown Dallas to get Patricia's PAP Scan and blood test. Those weeks just seem to drag along. We could not wait to go get her PAP Scan to see where we were at. We both were hoping to see that the test comes back positive. Patricia's pain medication was starting to run low. It is the same prescription that Dr. "O" had wrote for Patricia last time we were in to see him.

I called Dr. "O's" receptionist at the clinic and explain to her how Patricia's pain medication was running low and she only had like three pills left. The receptionist was telling me that the prescription was for 60 pills and there should still be 20 left. I explained to her I don't know how that could be. I've only been given her one for every four hours for her pain. The bottle only has three pills left. I tried to tell her I could not explain it but I do know that Patricia is going to need some more pain pills and we would not have enough to make it through the weekend. This was on a Thursday. The receptionist tells me that she would have to talk to Dr. "O" and if he wrote a prescription, it would be tomorrow morning.

After I got off the phone I got to thinking there's no way that there is supposed to be 20 pills left. I have been doing an outstanding job of keeping up with Patricia's medication and her time she supposed to take them. I would have never thought of to count the pills in the bottle. I know one thing, there were not 60 pills in the bottle, there's no way.

With Hospice we would just have to call and Patricia would have the pain pills the same day or the next. I guess we were getting pretty spoiled when Patricia was on Hospice. I was just making sure that I was staying on top of everything and all of Patricia's appointments. I was making sure Patricia would get all of her medications when she was supposed to. All I know is that Patricia will be out of pills by Monday.

The next morning, Patricia and I got up early and had our coffee together. We sure do enjoy our coffee. Then I made us some homemade biscuits and gravy with scrambled eggs. There's nothing like a good breakfast to start the day. I told Patricia I was going to run over to the clinic in Dallas to pick up her pain medicine prescription. As soon as I got back over here close to town I would run up to the pharmacy and get it field. I did not want Patricia to be worried about anything especially running out of pain medication. I have not heard back from the doctor's receptionist yet but I was not waiting.

After I arrived at the clinic I went up to the nurse's station desk and asked if there was a prescription for me to pick up for Patricia, her pain medication from Dr. "O." They sent me back to talk to Dr. "O's" nurse and she tells me again that Dr. "O" will not write a prescription because Patricia should still have more pills left. I showed her the bottle had 2 pain medicines left in it. She asked me to wait in the lobby because Dr. "O" was with another patient right now and when the Dr. was done he would come out in the lobby to speak with me.

I guess 10 minutes had gone by. I got up when I saw Dr. "O" coming into the lobby to meet him halfway with his nurse right behind him. She pointed me out and sternly said, "HERE HE IS!" and before I could say anything, he says, "I am not writing Miss. Fraley another prescription. I am not going to lose my license." I tried to explain to Dr. "O" that I am Patricia's caregiver at home and I have been very careful of dealing out her prescriptions on time and never had any problems like this before. All I know is that there are only three pills left and Patricia was going to run out of these pain pills before the weekend was over. The doctor tells me again, there is supposed to be 60 and there is no way she could be out and he will not write another prescription. Then he just turned around and walked away.

Man I cried all the way home thinking, what we are going to do now. Patricia is running out of pain pills. That is just what we need. I got to thinking maybe the pharmacy accidentally put 40 in the bottle instead of 60, which could be the only explanation. I went straight up to the pharmacy and explain to them how we seem to be short 20 pain pills. She tells me I just counted those this morning and that their count was right, the pharmacy could not explain it either. I am thinking this is not working! It is time to do something else quick.

Then I called the radiation doctor and asked him if he would mind seeing Patricia. She is having bad pain in her left leg and would he mind giving Patricia a prescription for pain pills. I told him how Patricia was running out and he said no problem. I will say it again that radiation doctor is all right in my book. If I was to give it my best guess, I think it was on the pharmacy. How I calculated that was when I brought the new prescription home with the new 40 count. I poured them into the 60 count bottle, looked in it, and I know that is where it was before when I picked up that bottle.

Next time I will count the pills. I am so glad all that worked out okay.

On 04/15/2015 is the morning Patricia has a 10 AM appointment at Baylor Texas Oncology in Dallas to have her X-Ray that's called a PAP Scan and blood test. This is how I put it in my journal. Dr. "O's" office called and moved Patricia's appointment up from the 27 to April 15, 2015 for today.

Patricia seems to have 102 fevers each morning. It seems to come on in the nighttime. Leg and foot swelling has gone away for four days. She has no pain in her hip and leg almost 5 days now. We are hoping to get more information from the test and the PAP Scan from today. We still do not know what is next, Patricia has been so strong. I admire her bright attitude. I love her so much! I pray to God the tests that are taken today are very positive.

The time is 6:05 AM and I hear Patricia waking up. She is not to eat this morning because of the PAP Scan that is scheduled for 10:30 AM this morning, and hoping for a good lunch maybe Burger King, and a good day. I was the first one up so I pushed the button on the coffee pot and got it started, then went in and sat with Patricia while we were waiting on the coffee to get ready. I guess the best part of waking up is Folgers in your cup. You know that's right. Patricia and I enjoy watching the sun coming up, the front of our house faces east and it is so beautiful to see the sun shine through the pine trees in the morning. Patricia and I would have some great conversations over coffee.

There were many mornings we felt that we were so blessed no matter what was going on. We both have the best attitude we possibly could. I can say one thing about Patricia, I think over the last six or seven months I've hardly heard Patricia complain maybe twice and it was very minor. She always stays positive. I admired her strength, her hope, and the love she always showed me with so many kind words.

Patricia could only have a few sips of coffee. Plus, she is not supposed to eat anything this morning but I think she was so excited about going to Baylor and getting some tests ran and get this PAP Scan. She was okay with that. I got all of our paperwork and Patricia's wheelchair loaded up into the pickup truck. When I came back to get Patricia she had already walked to the front porch. She never stops amazing me. She probably could have made it all way to the truck, but I went ahead and carried her out there. Patricia was getting that strong.

It took a little while driving around downtown Dallas but we finally found Baylor Hospital and where we were supposed to go in. We got there and checked in at the nurse's station. Patricia and I were noticing this little old lady who would go around and set with different people there in the waiting area. When they would get up to go back for their treatment she would go around, sit, and start visiting with somebody else.

After about five times she got around to us, she was asking how we were doing and how we looked like a wonderful couple. She said, "Is there anything I can pray for you about? Let me know?" We said, "Sure, we like prayer," so she said a little prayer with us. Then it was Patricia's time to go back for treatment. While I was getting Patricia already to go back, the little old lady gave Patricia this little red rose. Where she got it from, I do not know. We had been watching her for an hour. We never saw her give anyone else any roses. When she sat down with us, we did not see any roses in her hands. I think she was an Angel.

I will let the reader know right here that the picture on the front of this book is the picture I took of Patricia on 04/15/2015. You can see the hope, peace, and love in her eyes. God love her. Patricia was feeling pretty good that day. You can see the smile that is on her face.

The Nurse Technician came in and gave Patricia her radiation dye into her veins in her arm. She told Patricia she would have to set still for one hour so it could run all through your veins. It just so happened there was a little TV in the room so Patricia got to watch some of the Ellen DeGeneres show. That is one of Patricia's favorite shows.

The hour went by pretty fast. They came and got Patricia and took her back to get her PAP Scan ran. After we left the clinic, Patricia and I drove through a Jack-in-the-Box. Patricia got her a Jumbo Jack with cheese, some curly fries and a Sprite to drink. We just drove around the rest of the afternoon. It was a beautiful day.

Since Patricia now had a Medicaid card, we can still get home health care for her. I even talked to a physical therapist to see if they could come out and work with Patricia on some kind of physical therapy.

A very nice physical therapist came out to the house to visit with Patricia. We explained to her how we just got off Hospice and how it would be very beneficial for Patricia to start working out more to help strengthen her. The physical therapists showed Patricia some of the exercises that they would be doing. She visited with us for almost an hour. She could see in Patricia how eager she was to start working out. She explained to us that she would have to run it through Medicaid to make sure they were going to cover the costs and she would get back with us as soon as possible.

It has been nine months now since we found out Patricia has an inoperable tumor in her lower stomach. It's just after three days from April 15 and Patricia started having a little more pain in her right leg and lower back. We both were thinking and hoping that this is just temporary. Then after a few more days before her new appointment we found out the test results from the last appointment on the 15th were back.

I called Kristie the youngest daughter to see if she would like to come up to her mother's appointment on the 27th, that way we all could hear what Dr. "O" had to say about the results on Patricia's tests. Patricia and I were hoping so much that the test results were going to be positive.

The day of Patricia's appointment in April.

Today is Patricia's appointment on April 27, 2015. Patricia and I set out in the pickup truck, in the parking lot, just enjoying each other's company while talking, and waiting for Kristie to arrive. I remember telling Patricia, "You are all right in my book." I told Patricia, "I am going to write a book about you someday you are a very amazing woman." After Kristie showed up, we all went on in to Patricia's appointment.

We were on time for her appointment, that's just the way we roll. When Dr. "O" stepped into the room, I could tell by his face that the news was not looking good. He started explaining to us that the cancer Patricia has in her body has spread even more, it was in her liver, her lymph nodes, and even more into Patricia's lower spine. He felt at this time Chemo probably would not help Patricia much at this date.

That news broke my heart and Kristie's, too. It's like the air was sucked out of the room. That's the first time I have ever heard Patricia say I don't want to die. Patricia and Kristie started to cry. I looked at Dr. "O" and asked, "Is there anything we can do, maybe some low-dose chemo treatments? We need to try something." The Dr. explained it would probably make Patricia even sicker and that he would write Patricia a prescription for some morphine and some more hydrocodone for pain. He felt Patricia will need them moving forward. When Dr. "O" left the room, he had his nurse write up a prescription for Patricia.

I gave Patricia the biggest hug and told her, "It is not over yet and we are still in it to win it, my sweet love muffins." I also felt so bad for Kristie. That is not the news I was hoping for any of us to hear. I know Kristie loves her mother so much. They have always been so close. The whole time we were on our way home, Patricia and I would talk about how we are not giving up and how we still had the Lord on our side.

After we got home, I called the Healthcare Nurse to let her know about the results from the test and explained to her how the doctor sent us home with morphine. It looks like Patricia will be starting it today. The nurse came out to the house to explain how the morphine works. This was new to me. She explained to me how morphine tricks the mind and how it works to help relieve the pain on top of the other pain pill. I let her know how I felt about the morphine and how I wasn't really sure that Patricia was ready for morphine right now! Personally, I think they were overdoing it in the hospital with the morphine. Patricia's pain level was only#1 or#2 and the pain pills seem to be keeping it under control.

Our only concern was to keep Patricia pain free and as comfortable as possible. I will be sure to note it all in my log every day and keep a close eye on Patricia's symptoms. I was doing this, every day, and this is what I put in the

Journal on the third day of being on morphine. April 29, Wednesday, med's 7 AM one morphine 30 mg tablet, her temperature at 1 PM was 98.5. Blood pressure at 1 PM was 94/57, pulse 96. Temperature at 6:45 PM was 99.8. Medicine at 7 PM, took morphine and her pain number was #3. Blood pressure at 7 PM was 84/57, pulse was 107. That is a little high, Medicine at 7:30 PM, she took two sodium bi-carbonate, and one stool softener.

I was noticing by Friday that Patricia's hands would shake a lot. It was hard for her to hold her coffee cup and she seemed to be going into a comatose state. Patricia seemed to be getting weaker. I could just tell that Patricia was not being herself. I know Patricia pretty well and I know she would not like being in that state. I spoke with the Health Care Registered Nurse about maybe pulling Patricia back off the morphine and if it would be all right if we pulled back slowly on the doses, she agreed with me.

The next day on Sunday, we had one morphine in the morning at 7 AM and then morphine on Monday, May 4. I could already see an improvement in Patricia. This is what I wrote on that day, May 4, she took her medicine at 7 AM, she had one morphine and one hydrocodone, at 11 AM bowel movement, that's good.

Patricia started becoming herself again and also enjoys her coffee. Her shows came on TV and I just knew she wasn't ready for that morphine yet. I know she would've done the same for me. I was thinking the doctors sure are in a hurry to prescribe morphine. I just don't think Patricia was ready for that yet.

Here is Patricia's log for May 7. She took her medicine at 6 AM, one hydrocodone, at 8:30 we took her blood pressure, it was 76/46. Pulse 86, med's 10 AM one hydrocortisone. 11 AM one Tylenol, bowel movement, pain level at number two, that's great. Even that Friday was a great day. Patricia was laughing and had a great spirit about her.

I am still so admired by her strengths, her hope, and the joy in her heart for living. Patricia and I were living each day to the fullest.

Around May 15 on a Friday, I started noticing Patricia getting a little weaker. It was around this time I was really starting to get serious about starting a book. I know it was the Holy Spirit guiding me and I have such a big great desire in my heart to share the story about Patricia and her hope, her peace, and the love we shared together. I went out and bought a book that zips up and started writing things down. I would like to share some of these writings to help express my truest feelings for these days that I put on paper.

I am going to read right from my notes, starting 05/04/2015, it is 4 AM. I just carried Patricia from off of the couch and put her in the bed. Dr. "O" has put Patricia on morphine starting on 04/27/2015.

On that day, Dr. "O" tells us Patricia is diagnosed with Sigma Cell Carcinoma of the Cervix and it is spreading to her lower back bone of her spine. It is spreading and getting worse and the treatment is not going to do much good. Patricia and I are not giving up. God is still in control, and HOPE Is STILL ALIVE.

On May 5, Patricia is coming off the morphine. It was making Patricia not all here. This morning she is sitting up and more responsive. The registered nurse from hospice says that's okay let's wait on taking the morphine for now.

On 05/20/2015 this morning at 6 AM, we slept in. We both needed the extra sleep. Patricia was a lot clearer this morning. On the third day from getting off the morphine, Patricia and I was talking yesterday about the effects that the morphine was taking on her and how it put her in a state almost like a coma. She couldn't even take her medication and she stopped eating, smoking, and even put her in a state to not take a drink of water.   We talked about her not wanting to be in that state of mind. Patricia told me thank you so much and that she loves me with all her heart. I told Patricia, "You would have done the same for me."

Last night Patricia started to get her appetite back and ate a big piece of cheesecake with a big smile on her face. Just taking the hydrocodone seems to be enough to manage the pain. Patricia has had three bowel movements in the last two days after seven days of no bowel movements.

Patricia and I agreed on other types of pain management like pillows under her legs, sitting up in her wheelchair, leg exercises, and a vibrator to rub on her leg where the sciatic nerve has been giving her trouble. All that combined, seems to be working just fine. We are just glad for her to be off morphine.

Patricia still has her dignity, her hope, and her love. She still has her thoughts and a voice while still having a quality of life. Plus, she enjoys watching The Big Bang Theory, NCIS and her soaps, drinking coffee and so much more.

Kellie came over today and visited with her mother while I went to do a job down by Eureka and then go by the shop in Kearns. I had to turn in some invoices and pick up a check. That's our Kellie! She was always there when we needed her. God bless her. I called Patricia at 12:30, she answered the phone and I was able to talk to Patricia and let her know I would be home in 45 minutes. Patricia sounded good and clear and told me to be careful and that she loves me. That was so sweet to hear to my ears. If Patricia had been on the morphine, I would have missed that. I love Patricia and I know she would have done the same for me, THAT'S LOVE! This is what I wrote on 05/15/2015, it went like this. I need to go back and talk about Mother's Day.

On 05/11/2015, what a great day, all the girls came over Kellie, Kristie, Katie and Melinda with all six of our grandchildren. Starting from the oldest to the youngest, Aubrey, Layeh, D'Amari, Emily, Nicholas and Ava, she's the baby. Katie was the first to arrive. She brought a rose and a dinner for her mother. Patricia was in great spirits, laughing and had a great visit with all of us. God is good. I know God has Patricia in his hands. Praise God it was such a great blessing to see Patricia enjoy her Mother's Day :-)

Back to 05/15/2015, it is 10 AM Friday morning. I just can't seem to get comfortable enough to leave Patricia alone for more than an hour at a time. It's been three weeks since Patricia has been able to get up on her own and walk. Patricia did get up yesterday morning from the bed to her walker five times, it's so important that Patricia tries to keep her strength up. I also tell Patricia how important it is to drink more water and move as much as she can. She has more pain in her lower back then in her leg. I am so hopeful she can get the will to work out her muscles more and get stronger.

I called in yesterday to Dr. Kroger to set up her next appointment for May 27, to change out Patricia's nephrostomy tubing's, it is time. I also would like to mention that Dr. "O" has sent Patricia home two times now with just pain control. Patricia has such a strong will to get better and I hear Patricia praying to the Lord for strength and healing. Patricia has a "Don't quit," attitude like no one I have ever met. I love this woman with all my heart. She is the love of my life and God has put us together at this time to be a blessing to one another that I know. I pray each day to Jesus for the restoring of Patricia's body and to remove all the sickness and diseases from her. I know he is with her. That gives me peace and hope. Oh, and so much joy, that is my strength.

On 05/16/2015, I had to make the call this morning to tell the hospice registered nurse that I feel Patricia is getting weaker, and has not eaten in two days. It's hard for her to swallow, even to drink water. I asked the registered nurse, "What do we do from here?" The nurse tells me she feels that Patricia needs to get the liquid morphine started. I told the nurse Patricia is not in much pain. She sleeps a lot and seems to be comfortable.

I called Patricia's oldest daughter Kellie to let her know. That was a hard phone call to make, let me tell you. Patricia's younger daughter Kristie text me to say she was scared. I text Kristie back and said, "Have no fear the Lord is near." God love her. I have been thinking of the title for my book. I feel it is time to get Patricia's story out. My first title was going to be "Holding Patricia's Hand," but I decided to go with "Patricia's Voice." Patricia had to go back on hospice.

Patricia went back on Hospice

Now this is what I wrote down for 05/19/2015, Patricia had a big piece of chocolate cake last night after helping her to get to the bed, hospice delivered yesterday. I know it might be the last time we have to move off of the couch. Patricia really liked her cake and milk.

Patricia's friend Miss Rita just came by to say hi. Miss Rita is the sweet lady that was coming out to see Patricia the first time we were on hospice but she no longer worked for that company. She keeps in touch with Patricia either calling, or texting, they had become pretty good friends with one another over these last few months.

Miss Rita says that she can see the change in Patricia and she wanted to let me know that she has never seen a man that takes as good of care of his wife as much as I do. She has been in healthcare for over 25 years. That was a great compliment, I needed that. Patricia just wakes up and says to Miss Rita, "Jimmy's getting the cookies". Miss Rita asked me who's Jimmy. I was a little puzzled. I got to thinking that Patricia told me once when she was in grade school. Her first boyfriend was named Jimmy. Maybe it was a memory back from a party they were going to have at school. It was such a blessing. Miss Rita came by to visit with Patricia. She said a prayer over both of us. God love her.

I just started Patricia on the oral solution of the morphine. I know Patricia's pain is increasing. My best friend and the love of my life, it is so hard for me to see Patricia this way after 21 years together. There is no one like my Patricia, it is 1:30 PM and I am crying like a baby. Starting this morphine is like, it's time. It hurts way down inside. If you can see the teardrop stains on this paper, just know how far they had to travel. I just gave Patricia her morphine by syringe. I can barely sit here and write this. I told

Patricia just how much that she means to me and that she is my best friend in the whole world. She is the love of my life, my love muffin, my sunshine, and I will be here to hold your hand. This hurts, sorry for the teardrop stains. I hope this doesn't smear. It's time to suck it up and get back to work.

On 05/20/2015, there is so much more to know about Patricia but for this book, it is a story of a woman that was in it to win it. Living day by day, Patricia's fighting spirit was full of positive attitude and lots of it. Its 1:20 PM, I am sitting here at Patricia's bedside. She is in a deep rest. Her breathing is getting lighter. I know Patricia can hear me so I just keep talking to her. I am saying over and over that Katie loves you, Kristie loves you, Kellie loves you, Melinda loves you, and I love you. You are the love of my life. Jesus loves you and when I told Patricia my mother really loves you, she opened her eyes a little bit.

Now this is what I wrote for 05/21/2015. This morning I woke up at

6 AM, just having 4 and a half hour of sleep and grab some coffee. Patricia wakes up to me praying to Jesus and asking him to fill her body with healing. Patricia gives me this big smile. I gave Patricia some cool coffee into a straw. Patricia drinks it right down five or six sips, then Patricia opened her eyes and says good morning and that she loves me.

After last night I was so happy to see her alert and loving to me. When I leaned over to kiss Patricia on the four head, she wrapped her arms around my neck and pulled me down to her and gave me the biggest hug. That warmed my heart. To my surprise Patricia said I can't stay in the bed all day and that she wants to go to the living room. I said, "GREAT!" I carried her to the couch.

Friday, on 05/22/2015 at 12:05 PM the Chaplain just left. He came by to pray with Patricia and me. Patricia is in almost like a comatose state. I know she hears us. God love her. I would like to stop right here for just a little bit.

Today is 08/20/2015 and it falls on a Thursday. The time is 11 AM I woke up this morning with such a strong desire to finish the story about my best friend Patricia. I started writing in this book at 6:30 AM this morning and enjoying my coffee and reflecting on what all I have written up to this point. It is raining, it's sure nice to see the rain, and it has been 39 days since we had rain here in Texas, at least in this area anyway. I have just got back from taking a break, I went to town to get me a breakfast burrito and when I came back into the house I could smell Patricia in the air. I just don't know why, maybe it's the rain. It was raining at the point of this story about the love of my life. Maybe it's her way of letting me know, we got this. I know I am a plumber but this leaking coming from my eyes, I cannot fix it. Okay I got this, back to the story.

I had called the girls the night before to let them know the condition their mother was in, that is a hard phone call to make. It breaks my heart for the girls to see Patricia in this condition, the girls and I stepped out onto the front porch. We had the most regretted conversation. We talked about funeral arrangements for Patricia.

I really admire how all of us came together with making the arrangements. All of us decided when the time would come that we would just have Patricia cremated and all the girls were okay with that. They said they had conversations in the past with their mother, and said she did not have a preference. We also discussed what we would do with Patricia's ashes. The girl's first idea was to take her out to the lake and spread her ashes around the lake area. Then we talked about maybe getting an urn and one of us keeping ashes at their house. Then we discussed maybe getting a weeping willow tree and putting Patricia's ashes under a tree in the front yard. Then I told them of an idea that I had about getting a rosebush and putting Patricia's ashes under the rosebush out in the rock garden right under the three-tier cast-iron lamppost.

I feel that Patricia would have liked that idea. She loves it here so much, all of us agreed on that idea. That conversation went very well. I had already talked to a funeral home out in Quitman two weeks earlier and had the arrangements all set up just in case we needed their services. Sleep tight my love.

On 05/21/2015, it is hard for Patricia to swallow her pain pill so I have had her on that liquid morphine for four or five days now. I have to administer it through a syringe under her tongue, 25 mg per hour, we stop at 11 PM. She sleeps through the night pretty good. I know Patricia's time is close now. It's not that I don't have hope. Lord knows I have never lost it, and I know it is not for me to decide, that is for the Lord and his plans. It's now 11 PM, I just checked on Patricia, she is in a deep sleep, her breathing is shallow and she is in no pain. I sit at Patricia's bedside as much as I can, and talk to her. I know she can hear me.

Sometimes she raises her eye brows just to let me know. With the morphine in her system, it makes her pretty drowsy.

It's Friday, Memorial Day weekend on 05/22/2015, there has been so much rain water everywhere. I put all the little flags out front. There must be 25 of them. I am hoping Patricia may wake up and look out the window and see them. She likes having them out on holidays like this Memorial Day weekend.

It's 9:15 AM, I have been sitting here with Patricia this morning, drinking coffee and talking to her, letting her know how much she is loved. I would keep saying over and over that all the girls love you, all the grandkids love you, and Jesus loves you for the Bible tells you so, her breathing is getting so slow. She is hot to the touch. I have been putting cold rags on her to cool her down, it's helping. I can't get her to wake up. It's 9:30 AM, I have Kelly and Michael on the TV, she likes that show.

On Saturday, 05/23/2015, its 10:15 AM in the morning, the girls came by yesterday, Mindy, Kellie, Katie and Kristie. Patricia was in a comatose state all day. Her breathing was light and it's been going on three days with no water. We all was around Patricia's bed crying our eyes out playing Michael Bolton for Patricia, hoping it would maybe open her eyes and also to see Patricia smile. All of us were hurting. Patricia's older sister Sharon came by late this evening to visit with Patricia when I said to Patricia, your sister Sharon is here to see you. Patricia opened her eyes real big almost 20 seconds, she really loves her sisters. I am so glad they had a good visit together. I know Patricia could hear her. She would raise her eyebrows when Sharon would speak to her. God love her.

After everyone had left, it was close to midnight before I gave Patricia her last dose of the morphine, 25 mg in a little syringe under her tongue. I made a place to sleep on the floor next to her bed. I woke up from one little moan from

Patricia so I sprang to my feet to see if she was okay. She was okay. You see, I fell asleep last night praying for Patricia. To my surprise Patricia had her eyes open, the first thing I asked her was, "Would you like some water?" She said, "Yes please!" I can see when the morphine wears off a little bit.

She's more aware, she drank maybe 3 ½ straws full of water. I was so happy to see her get some water in her. Patricia was pretty hot with fever. I got some cold rags, five of them and moved them around her body. The fever broke in 30 minutes. That was great. Patricia did a few leg exercises for almost an hour. Patricia got to take one of her hydrocortisone pain pills crushed up in a spoon of water. I am wondering maybe if we should cut back on the morphine or not? I went outside to get some air. I can still see Patricia through the window. She was waving at me with the biggest smile. It melted my heart. I still know to this day that was Jesus, he gave me that moment and I'll cherish it forever. Patricia is so strong I

just have to thank Jesus. It's a good day
:-)

www.EricRoberts-Author.com

The day the love of my life left her body and her spirit went to be with Jesus.

Sunday, on 05/24/2015, this is exactly how I wrote it in my journal for that day. It goes like this, today is the day the love of my life left her body and her spirit went to be with Jesus. I woke up this morning at 5:30 AM. I had fallen asleep on the couch last night around 12:30.

When I first woke up, I went into the room to check on Patricia. I was relieved to see she was still breathing pretty well. So I went to start the coffee pot. It's slow. At 5:45 AM, I looked back in on Patricia and still seem to be resting well. I was standing at the coffee maker praying, asking God to let this be a good day and thanking Him for being in control. I had one cup of coffee at the kitchen table for it was five minutes till six. I got Patricia's morphine ready in the syringe that I had to put under her tongue. Patricia was still not swallowing very well. I walked into the bedroom with the coffee cup in one hand and her pain medicine in the other. Patricia was gone. No breathing at all. I knew right away she had passed. My heart is hurting so much. The love that we have shared over the last 21 years on this earth is over. It's so sad.

It is 9:45 PM I have so much more to say but I need to get some sleep. I am exhausted. It was just last night I started to write this book. This is a story that needs to get out there. I am going to title it Patricia's Voice. IT'S TIME! Good night my love I will see you in heaven. This is where I will have to leave this diary and move this story to my book. I GOT THIS.......... Do not harden your heart :-) :-) :-)

I would like to give a big thanks to the Hospice Healthcare Team that was helping me with Patricia's healthcare. It was 6 AM when I had called hospice to let them know that Patricia has passed away, and I also called all the girls. All I could say is your momma is gone to be with Jesus and she's okay. I went back into room to sit with Patricia and I held her hand and told her Jesus got this. She looks so peaceful and calm. One of my first thoughts was it sure would have been nice if Patricia could have had those nephrostomy tubes taken out of her back four months earlier. To Patricia that was her biggest challenge. God love her.

The Hospice Nurse arrived in 20 minutes to the house. The Nurse was so polite and caring after she looked in on Patricia. She made the phone call to the funeral home in Quitman. The Hospice Nurse even asked me if I would like for her to brush Patricia's hair to help make her look nice. That was so thoughtful of her. All the girls arrived at the same time. They all rode in one car. IT'S A SAD, SAD MORNING. We all know we are going to miss Patricia, but we will see her again someday in heaven.

A man was there from the funeral home to pick Patricia's body up by 10 o'clock. I do know in my heart that was just Patricia's body and her spirit has left to go be in heaven. You know, PATRICIA

WAS IN GOD`S HAND`S THE WHOLE TIME. It is a divine peace that surpasses all understanding. One of mine and Patricia's sayings was we like easy.

I would like to say to all the girls IF they are still reading this book by this time, LOL, just how much I love their mother. From the first day I met her, I was there to never ever let her stumble and fall. That hope, peace, love and caring heart that their mother showed is like NO OTHER. I wanted to thank Kristie, Katie, Kellie, and Melinda for their help and understanding through this great tragedy, I love them all. They are in my prayers every day.

This is a word from the author Eric Roberts, today is Friday, 08/21/2015, it has been three months since the love of my life and my soul mate passed away. I started writing this book about Patricia on 05/23/2015. It fell on a Saturday and I can only hope that it can express half of the experience Patricia had to endure in just nine months. God love her.

There is so much more to this story and I know if there are any healthcare workers out there that are taking care of a loved one, family member, or a good friend while working in the healthcare industry, my hat goes off to you. You know that person you are taking care of is your calling. That takes passion, humility, and a loving, caring heart to do what you are doing. From me to you, thank you for that and God bless you for it.

Never harden your heart, for Jesus will be there for your strength and your love and you're hope. You also have the Holy Spirit to help guide you and comfort you in all your ways. Again, thank you.

At this point, if there is still anybody reading this book I would like to share with you a few days after Patricia's passing and even some pictures. I can only pray I was able to express Patricia's Voice in the story. Now I would like to share with you some of what was in a diary, this is how it goes. Today I am starting a diary and a new chapter in my life without the best friend and love of my life.

Today is Wednesday, 05/27/2015, my love and inspiration passed away from cervical cancer. We found out Patricia Ann Kuempel / Fraley had a cancerous tumor in her cervix, then to find out two months after that, it was an inoperable cancer and spreading fast. From October 2014 to 05/24/2015 was just seven months, I am going to miss her smile, her inspiration, and her loving heart. It's time to drive on, rest in peace Patricia. 21 years.

Today is Thursday, 05/28/2015, the girls have been so helpful to me. I admire their strength at this so sorrowful time they all are so strong, just like their mother would have been. For me, it is just so hard to sit still for too long. I catch myself walking room to room. I think I have sat in every chair in the house and the front porch several times each, that's crazy huh?

The girls are doing such a great job of planning lots of details, some big and some small. I am so proud of them all. I know one thing, getting Patricia out of my conscious that is so hard. I love and miss her so much, so very, very much. I need to get this on paper before I break down and just cry. This afternoon, Mindy, Kristie, Katie, Kellie, two of the young grandchildren and me drove out to Quitman Texas to pick up Patricia's ashes.

After Patricia passed away last Sunday morning at 5:55 AM, Patricia stopped breathing she was in no pain. Hospice and the Funeral Home picked up Patricia and took her body away. I know her spirits in heaven with Jesus and I will see her again someday. Back to today, I will just have to get the whole story in my book called "Patricia's Voice."

Today after the girls and me, plus, the grandchildren picked up Patricia's ashes from the funeral home we went to a nursery and picked out a beautiful red rosebush, it's a Christian Dior. We brought it back to the house where we put some of Patricia's ashes under the rosebush that we all had picked out. We planted it in front of the house in the round rock garden with the three-tier lamppost.

Patricia loved it. She loved the beautiful front yard and loved living here. It took the four girls and 3 of the grandchildren to plant the rosebush, a real group effort. It was really, very nice. Tomorrow we are going to have a memorial service out in the front yard with friends and family. I am going to try to say what's in my heart tomorrow if I can keep from breaking down. I will give it my best shot I need to stop here. It's hard to. I have so much I need to get out there about a wonderful woman.

May 30th, Dear Journal, it's Saturday 7:15 PM, I just made myself eat. I even splurged and ordered Mexican food, which was great until I started eating it. Then here comes the tear crying over Mexican food. What's that about? Patricia got into my thinking. She loved to order from La

Pradera's Mexican food restaurant. We would always order beef enchiladas, our favorite and sweet tea with lemon.

I need to journal down all about a beautiful service that was held right here at the house Kellie and Alex came over earlier today. They planted some beautiful flowers in pots and arrange them real nice. We all worked so good together to see it is a carefree service. All the girls even gave the house a good old Oaky scrubbing, it sure needed it. Patricia would be so proud of how the girls came together and made it work. They made it as beautiful as possible. Shoot, I am proud of them.

We had 35 or so that could make it. Some just sent flowers and prayers, which we understand. Kristie and her boyfriend were so generous with drinks, ice, chips and a tablecloth and so much more, Kristie is so blessed. Katie made a wonderful picture sideshow of her mother from over the years and played music from her stereo, it was so nice of her. Melinda brought plates, snacks, and food.

Several people sent cards and flowers. We had them all arranged real nice out front on a little deck we built. This was to hold all the flowers. There were a lot of them. I had asked Mr. Donald, the Chaplain, to come out to pray with us. This is the same Chaplain that was with us when Patricia was on hospice the first time. He did know Patricia pretty well and knew that Patricia was safe with Jesus in his arms. We even had the grandchildren.

The Service started 5:30 PM. The weather was great and the yard was wet, but a nice day. The temperature was about 79°. If Patricia could have let us know, she would have been pleased. Kellie, Patricia's oldest daughter got up and shared with us the eulogy she had written a few days before. All the other three girls joined her. She did not want to speak alone. It was beautiful and she did an outstanding job so proud of them all.

I need to stop here, hoping to write some more in the book called "Patricia's Voice." Starting on chapter 3, I love you

Patricia ANN. I miss you so much, so very, very much. Your memorial service was carefree. I Love you :-) No worries. Say hi to Jesus and my mama for me. See you later. My eulogy for Patricia ANN read like this.

Eulogy For

Patricia Ann Fraley

By Eric Roberts

First I would like to thank all the girls and all the hard work they put into making this into a beautiful service. I know your mother would be so proud of all of you. Patricia, I like to call her Patricia ANN, the love of my life. I cannot think of a better place to honor Patricia's memories, then right here. She loves this place and all the smells, the fresh cut grass, the flowers, plus, these big old pine trees. Patricia has a lot of people who love her but I know Patricia is in heaven doing what she loves most, that is landscaping heaven, and I will see you later. I will miss you my love, my friend Patricia ANN. I was so blessed to know who you were, thank you. Love you, see you later.

Dear Journal. It is Sunday, May 31. It's been one week since the love of my life and my soul mate, not to mention my best friend in the whole world has passed. I miss Patricia so very much and I wish so deeply Patricia was here and healthy and I can see that smile that said no worries. I miss the joy she brought to our lives. It is a love affair that comes once in a lifetime and I am so blessed to know who Patricia was.

May God keep Patricia until I get to see her in heaven! I would love to hold Patricia's hand again and tell her I love you my love. No worries Patricia ANN! It is 11 AM Sunday morning. I got up at 5:30. I am almost back on a sleep schedule. I turned the lamppost off out front in the rock garden just at daylight. Patricia would have said its time to turn off the lamppost. One of us would have got it, most likely Patricia would have said, "I got this."

I just wanted to sit down for a minute and put in this book of Patricia's Voice, a Birthday Card that Patricia had picked out for me on my Birthday. Back on 01/01/2013, when I read it, I could feel

Patricia's presence and goose bumps all over my arms I would like to put it in the story and it goes like this.

> *You are the man for me. A loving birthday message from your wife, for one man can make me feel secure when he is by my side. One man conveys a quiet strength; his gentleness can't hide. One man holds for all ways my respect, my deepest pride. Only one man I have known you and you alone. One man's arms are warm enough to make a home for me. One man's touch can stir my heart and set my longings free. One man will be my love, my life for all eternity. One man has made my dreams come true, you and only you.*
>
> *Happy Birthday!*
>
> *With all my love, Patricia*
>
> *XX and OO*
>
> *Written by, Thomas Kincaid from Hallmark.*

It is now 11:45 AM and I am crying, I need to suck it up and drive on, that is what Patricia would have wanted. I may pack some things up but what's in my heart I will never give up. See you later Patricia love you and I will miss you for a very, very, very long time. :-)

Dear Journal it is Sunday and it is time to make the last part of this story, it has been a week now since my Love

Muffin passed away from this earth. I still find it hard to breath. I will go back to work tomorrow and try to let go of some of the hurt, but it is going to be hard. I will go on living in this world just knowing that I will always have been blessed to know Patricia and her love and memory will live on in my heart. Love you, my sunshine, see you again someday. Love always, Eric.

I would like to share some more of my journal with the reader if they could just hang with me, just a little longer. I will go through a few days of the journal on how I was feeling while writing this book and it goes on like this.

Monday, 06/01/2015, Dear Journal, its 7 PM got home from working, 2 service calls today. One was a gas test on a house, and cap off a fireplace. The other was just a sewer call. It was an easy day. I thought it might start getting easier letting my heart start to heal.

Wrong!!! At 4 o'clock, I was rolling around on the bed holding Patricia's pillow missing her so much. It is like I can hardly breathe, I just can't get the air to come into my lungs. I wish and hope I can relate to everybody I can, the true love Patricia and I were blessed to share on this earth. With Patricia not being here, it's like there is only half of me here left to figure out the rest of this story on my own. The pain in my heart is going to take a long time to heal, but you know I also know Patricia is with God. He's got this, I know it, too. I Love you Patricia Ann. I need to get into the book and go, go, go.

Thursday, June 4, Dear Journal, 12 days out from the day the love of my life has gone to be with the Lord. I got up this morning at 4:30. As soon as my eyes opened the first thing on my mind was Patricia. God I miss her so much.

I made my way to the coffee maker to push the button. Tearing up, I sure miss my coffee drinking friend. I mowed the whole yard yesterday thinking Patricia would love the way this place is looking. I cut up some trees that had fallen over from last Saturday's storm. I will keep this place looking good in honor of Patricia. That's what she would be doing if she was here. Patricia loved keeping our house and yard looking like this all the time. I will take a few good deep breaths and make my way through the day. It is supposed to get to 92° today, here comes the heat.

Friday, 06/05/2015, Dear Journal, it is 7 AM. I got up at 5 AM. I could almost hear Patricia saying push the button to start the coffee. Patricia is so much on my mind. God I miss her so much. Got the sheets and blankets off the bed and got them onto wash.

I can feel Patricia, it is time to turn the lamppost off, and it is getting light enough outside. I am just pacing back and forth on the front deck drinking my coffee looking out over the yard. With every step I think back 17 years ago when Patricia got me to drinking coffee. She got me taking a vitamin every morning, until then I had just been drinking Dr. Pepper's every morning and did not even like coffee.

After making coffee every morning for Patricia for two years, I had to give in and began to like it. Not bad, waiting until I was nearly 34 years old before I started drinking coffee. It is almost 7:30 AM, I need to put the clothes in the dryer and get going. It is still hard to believe Patricia is in heaven, I miss you.

June 7, Sunday, Dear Journal, it`s been two weeks since my heart was broken. I still am so lost without my love, my other half. I can't believe Patricia is not here this Sunday morning having coffee with me. She would enjoy listening to the birds while having the front door open, letting the house air out from the morning breeze. I can still feel her thoughts saying good morning my love. It's a beautiful morning and it is time to turn off the lamppost and what is for breakfast?

This life and this love we had with each other, comes along once in a lifetime. That is what gives me strength and my beliefs in our Lord and Savior. I believe with all my heart and soul that Patricia is in heaven. I need not be selfish. Thank you Journal for listening to me talk to you, it helps a lot. I pray every day that the Lord will help me get through the day. I still pray that the Holy Spirit will guide my way where it is a beautiful day and here is where my heart will stay. HEY, I am a poet and didn't even know it, LOL.

Dear Journal, it's me again, it was a nice day. I got a lot of mowing done today. At 4:30 PM, I was sitting out on a lawn chair in the front yard looking at how really nice the yard looks. There are times Patricia is on my mind and I just had to break down and cry. I miss Patricia so very, very much. It is still hard to breathe. I just cannot believe she is gone. I love her so much.

June 9, Dear Journal, 15 days out from the day Patricia, the love of my life, left this earth to go be with the Lord. It hurts so much. I cry every day. It is 7

Author Eric E. Roberts

AM. I got up at 4:30 AM this morning made my way to the coffee pot to push the button. Oh God, I miss Patricia so very, very much. I miss her smile, her caring heart, her touch, her laughter and so many little things.

I got all the plants and flowers watered, talked to the rosebush that we planted in Patricia's honor. It's so lonely not having her here. I am even crying over my breakfast. It is so sad. I just cannot get over Patricia not here. I still wander through the house room to room. I know she is with Jesus and I have to get my joy from that.

I know if Patricia was here right now she would say it's time to turn the lamppost off and the yard looks so beautiful. I could hear her say I love you with all my heart. I really miss that, and so much more. I love you Patricia ANN, I know I will see you again someday. The first thing I am going to say to Patricia ANN is thank you for loving me, see we got this.

June 17, Dear Journal, 24 days out and it is raining this morning. I got up this morning at 5 AM holding Patricia's pillow a little tighter last night. I push the button on the coffee maker. I sit out on the deck listening to the rain hitting the tin cover over the deck drinking my coffee thinking about Patricia. I sure am missing her so much, I broke out in not just a cry but I broke out into a full out bawling. I think it is the first deep, deep cry that I have had so far. Not for me but for Patricia. I feel so bad she got sick. My heart hurts for her. Crying out to God that I just need to believe Patricia is with Him and she's okay God has got this.

I know I should not worry, I know my faith should comfort me, but it still hurts so much. I sure miss my sweet, sweet love, the love of my life my soul mate. I don't know if I will cry every day. I just know Patricia is still in my heart, the love of my life and there is a big hole in my heart. It is time to dry my eyes and my runny nose and keep believing in God's grace, knowing God is still in control and the Bible is true. I will see my love again someday in heaven. I love you Patricia, see you again someday.

Sunday, June 21, good morning Journal, I was just out on the front deck talking to the Lord and thanking Him for keeping Patricia in His hands. It still hurts each time I think about Patricia getting sick. It is such a great tragedy to not have her to share the company. We shared everything with each other. I miss my love muffin so much. A woman like Patricia comes along only once in a lifetime. She is to me, truly a lady. Currently, the lamppost is on, I turned it off and making coffee, pushing the button on the coffee maker each day. I know she will always be a part of the rest of my life. She will be a part of my memory of the love I shared with my soul mate. Patricia and I will hold onto her precious memory, as long as God is willing.

Today is the fifth Sunday since Patricia has gone to be with Jesus. It still takes my breath away. Sometimes it is hard to believe she's still not here, today is Father's Day. It is 7 AM, who knows, I might just go fishing. I need to dry my eyes and thank Jesus for all my girls and grandchildren. I know God is still in control. I am surely blessed. It is time to turn the lamppost off, write to you later. Love you Patricia Ann.

Author Eric E. Roberts

Independence Day

Today is 07/04/2015, Dear Journal, I cannot believe it's already July 4. It is 5:30 AM, I got up early this morning, and I woke up at 4:30 AM. I did fall asleep last night around 9:30, I have been working pretty hard on the yard, wanted it to look good for the Fourth of July. The flags are out down the front of the yard. The rosebush has five or six blooms coming out and the yard is green. The yard looks really nice. I just came in from off the front deck.

I had to cry this morning thinking of just how much I miss Patricia, the love of my life, thanking God for giving me the time I had with her. I would talk to the Holy Spirit thanking him for being there with me and giving me the strength and guidance and peace.

Tomorrow would be mine and Patricia's 21st anniversary. Twenty-one years together, I am sure going to be missing

Patricia and her being here for this one. We were looking forward to the big 21 years. Well, Journal, I will get off here it is sad, but I will make it through with Christ who strengthens me. Love you Patricia ANN. 21 years :-)

07/04/2015, Hi Journal, it is me again it is 12:45 PM and here I am crying again. My heart aches so much. I miss my Patricia Ann and yearn so much to hold her. What got me to crying was that I just had to read what I wrote this morning. I am trying so hard, but the love we had shared together was so real and so unconditional. IT IS RARE!!

The last three years we spent together was more than one word could ever describe. I just know that Jesus got a great woman in heaven and He is keeping Patricia for me. I will always keep my trust in the Lord. That gives me my Hope Joy, and Peace. I thank God every day for His grace, and I am staying positive. I will stop here for now. Good night Patricia, sleep tight and just remember always I love you. Patricia will always have a place in my heart and thank you so much. I will see you again someday. I will stop writing this story now and hope you will enjoy the pictures in the back of this book. Thank you for reading this true story about Patricia. I hope her voice will be an inspiration to someone that finds their self in a situation similar to this.

The End

Written By

Eric E. Roberts, Author

About the Author

Eric E. Roberts wanted to write a book for over 30 years. Now finally at 55 years old, Eric has written his first book and for it to be a "True Story," was a great challenge for him. A Licensed Plumber by Trade, Eric has always felt that becoming an Author was an accomplishment that required a College Degree. Moving from school to school as a kid in his early years created many learning challenges that resulted in inadequate reading and writing skill sets. At the age of 22 Eric earned his General Equivalency Diploma. It was an encouragement to accomplish this and the result sparked his desire to write a book.

Thankfully, he had a Mother who raised him in Church and taught him about the Lord and the Holy Spirit, which gave him strength to draw from and in turn played a huge roll in leading him to seek other ways to further his education. He later joined the U.S. Army at the age of 30 years old, to "Be all he could be in the Army!" While serving in the military, Eric took college courses in Criminal Law and Criminal Justice. Six years passed quickly in the service and Eric soon received requests to return home where his presence was required full time.

The desire to write a book was strong and steadily tugged on his heart, but what to write and how was still a mystery! After all these years Eric had no idea what he could write about. Up to this point, he had reading and writing disabilities that he still needed to overcome in order to write a book for others to read, he thought.

Several more years passed and the desire to write was still there but seemed that his dream may never be reached. Then all of a sudden on January 13th, 2015, while accompanying his wife Patricia during a stay at the hospital for medical tests to be performed on her, the idea for Eric's book was revealed to him. He decided to write from inspiration of the medical events surrounding Patricia and the care she was receiving from her Healthcare Providers. Eric realized his wife was in the battle for her life and he needed to be a voice for her. He would write his book and title it, "Patricia's Voice, Hope-Peace-Love."

How was the next step to be solved? A Friend suggested Speech to Text Software and a computer! That idea really changed the playing field. Finally, for Eric, the dream to write a book was achievable and necessary.

Patricia's Album

Moments In Time

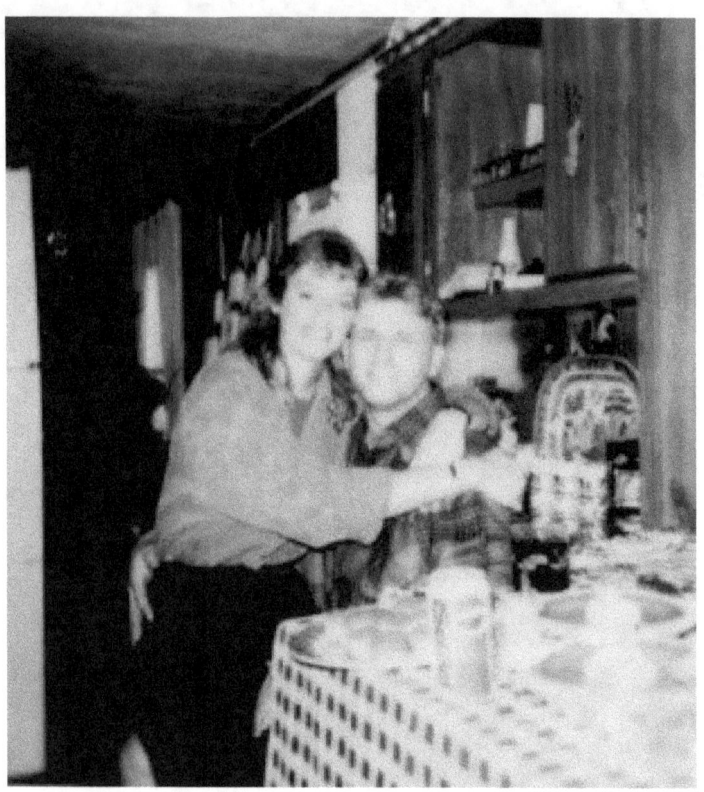

This is Patricia and I, in 1994. Our first Thanksgiving together! We look so happy....

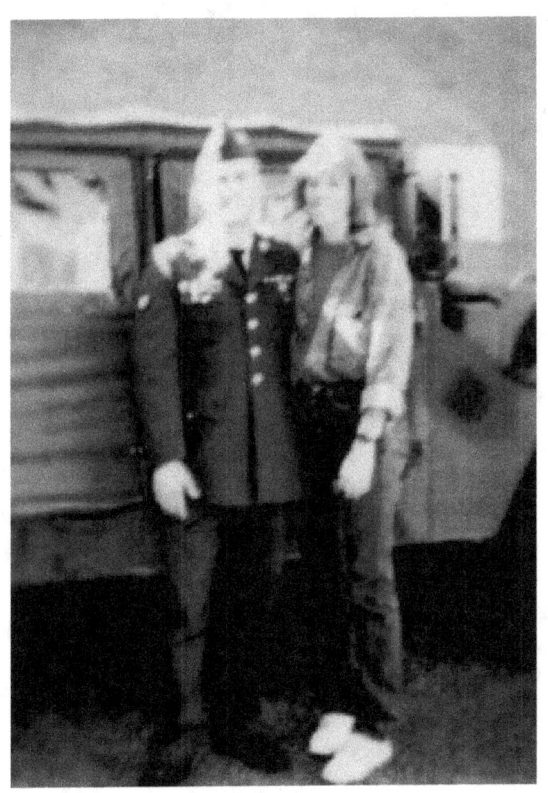

This picture was taken on the day that Patricia and the girls came out to my army unit and had Christmas dinner.

Author Eric E. Roberts

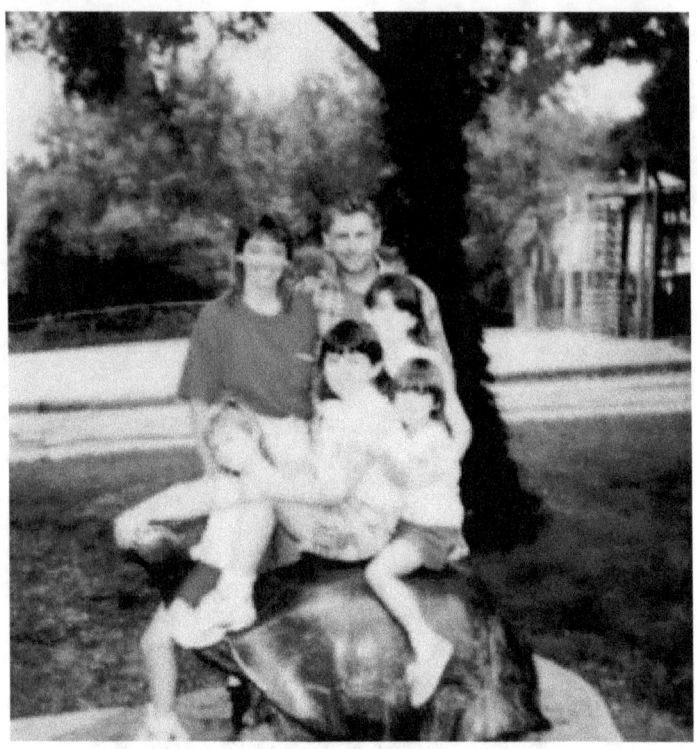

This is a picture of Patricia, the girls and I celebrating Easter at the Dallas Zoo.

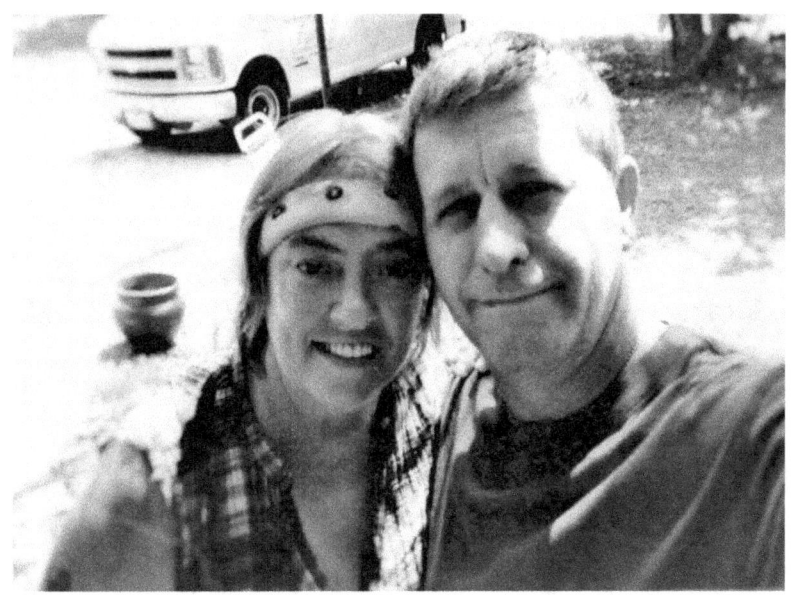

This is a picture of Patricia and, I
that was taken about a year before
she got sick with the cancer.

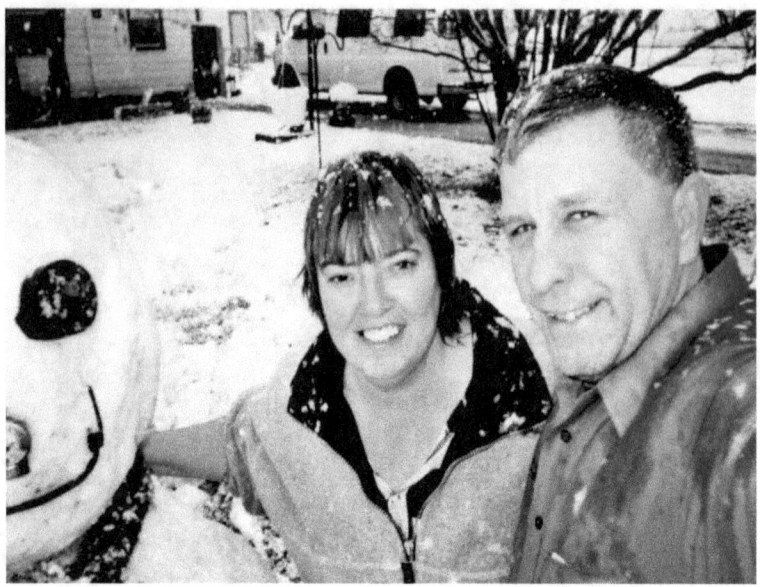

This is a picture of Patricia and me
with the Snowman that we built.
You can see the pride in our faces.

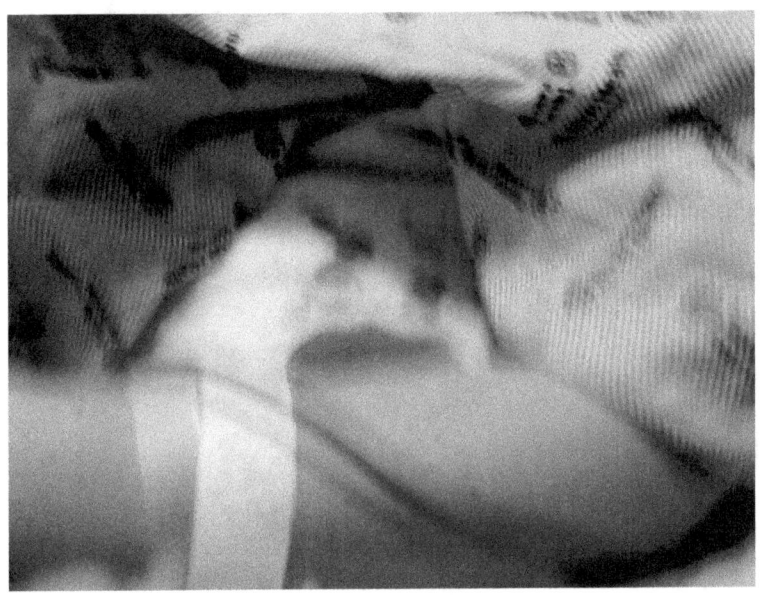

This is a picture of Patricia's blood transfusion leaking on the pillow our first night there in ICU.

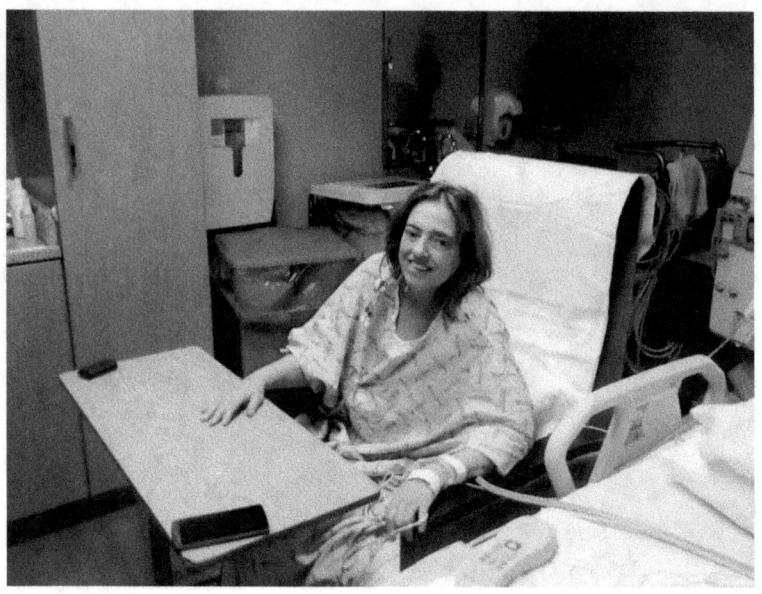

This is a picture of Patricia in ICU at
Presbyterian Hospital. I was so glad
to see her sitting up.

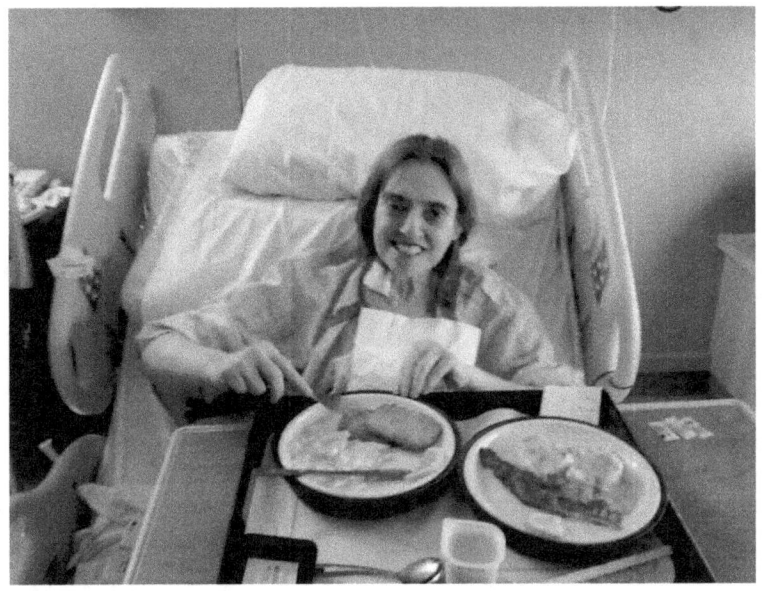

This picture was taken right after
they moved Patricia up to her own
room on the sixth floor. You can see
the smile on her face from all the
good food. God bless her!

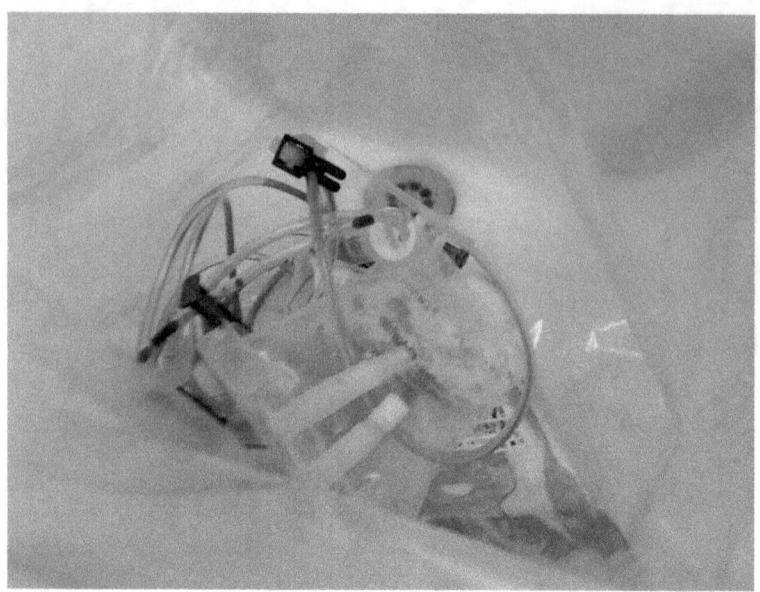

This is a blood transfusion bag that
they had put in the sink in our room.
It was supposed to go right into a
Bio-Trash Can.

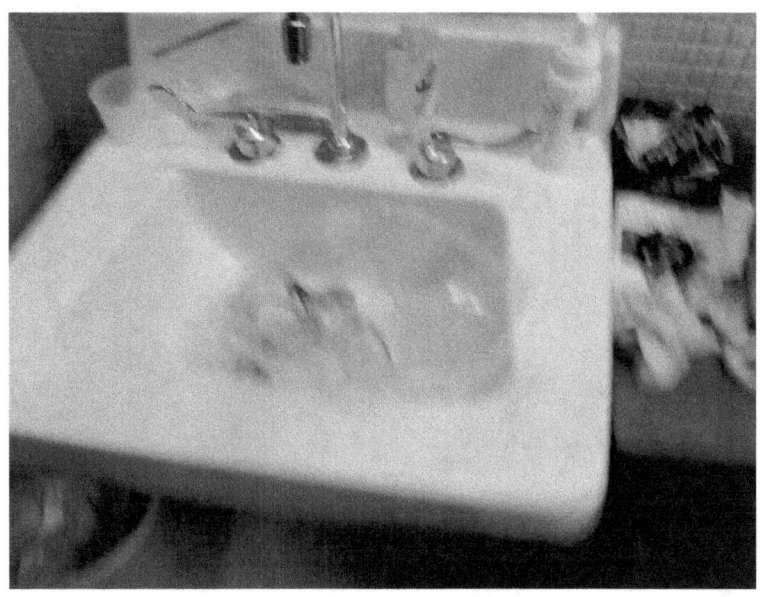

This is the sink in Patricia's room. You see our personal items on the back of the sink.

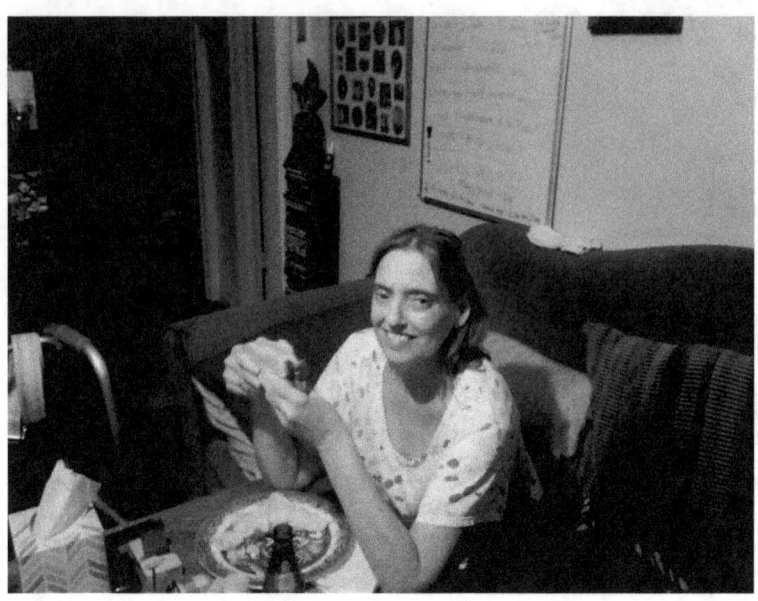

This is Patricia enjoying her lunch at
the house, always positive, always
smiling.

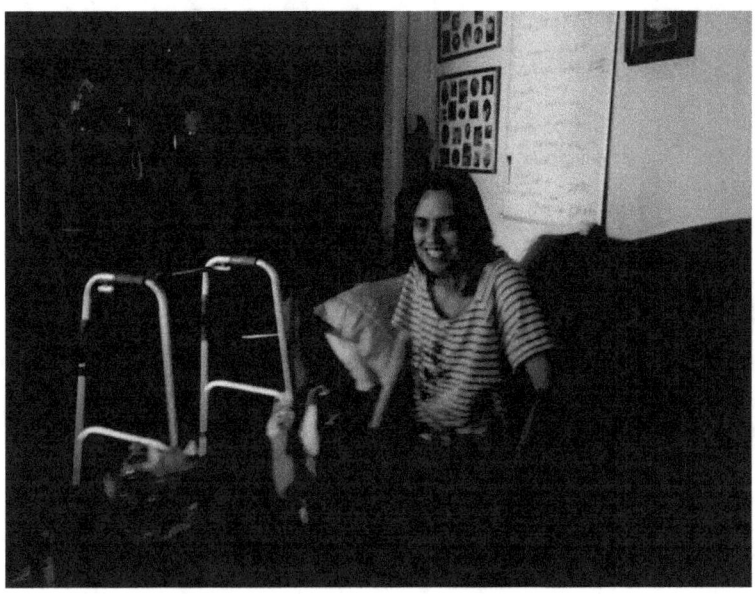

Patricia on a good day. We had just gotten home from seeing the kidney specialist. He was telling us that Patricia's kidneys are doing fine.

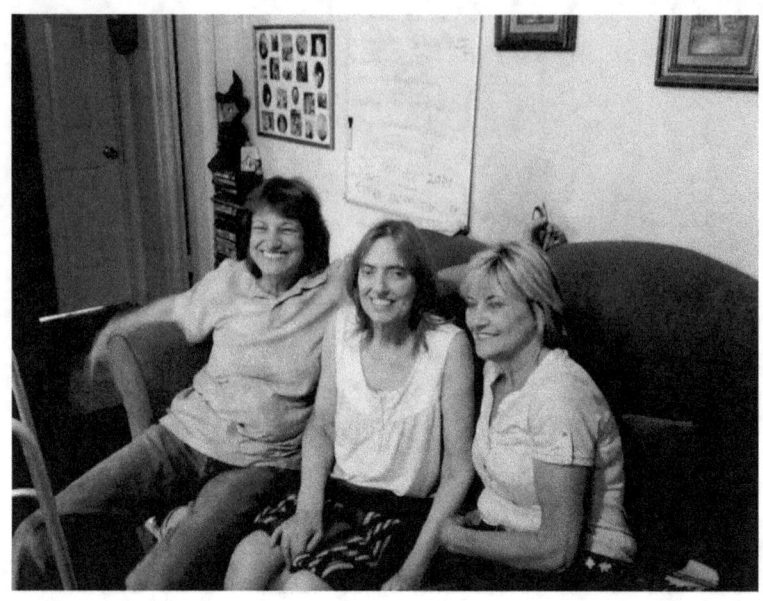

One afternoon, Patricia was enjoying the company of her two sisters, Sharon and Karen.

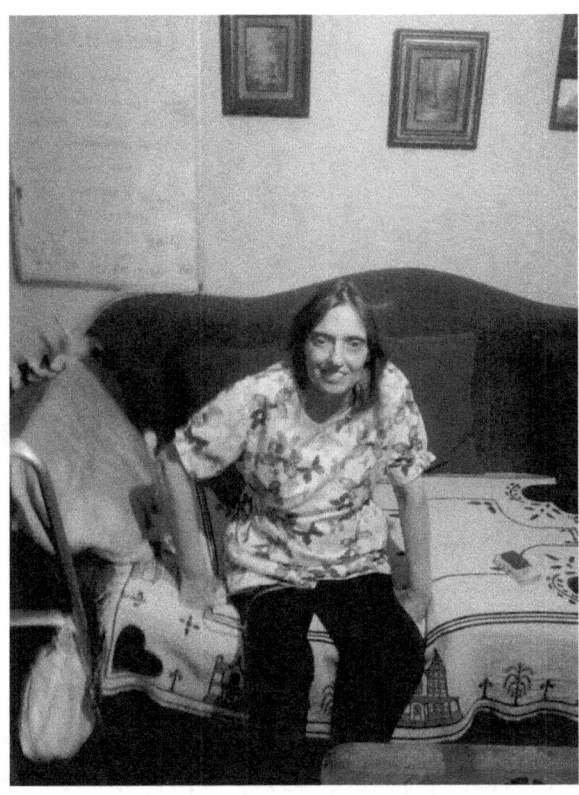

This is the morning Patricia and I were getting ready to leave to go to Parkland Hospital. The day started out great but ended up disappointing.

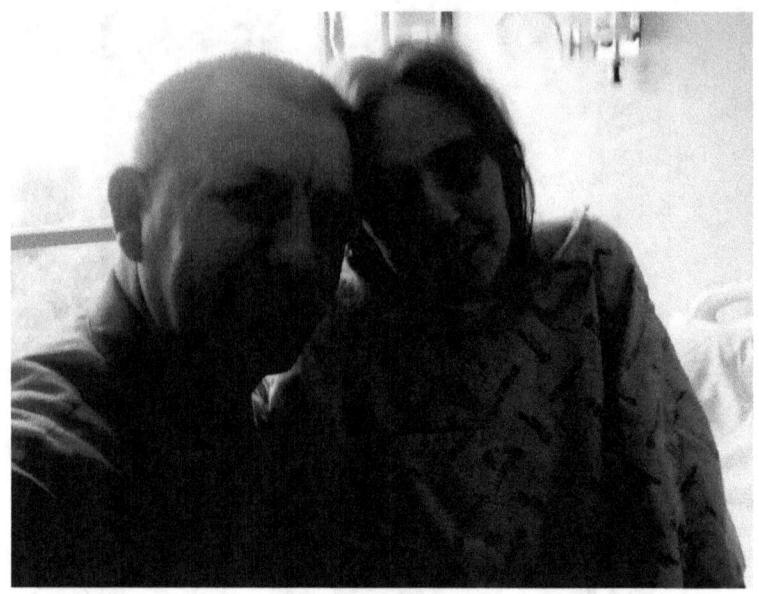

There's a good-looking couple, the second time we were back up at the hospital to finally get some radiation treatments. Patricia still hadn't received her yellow gown after eight days.

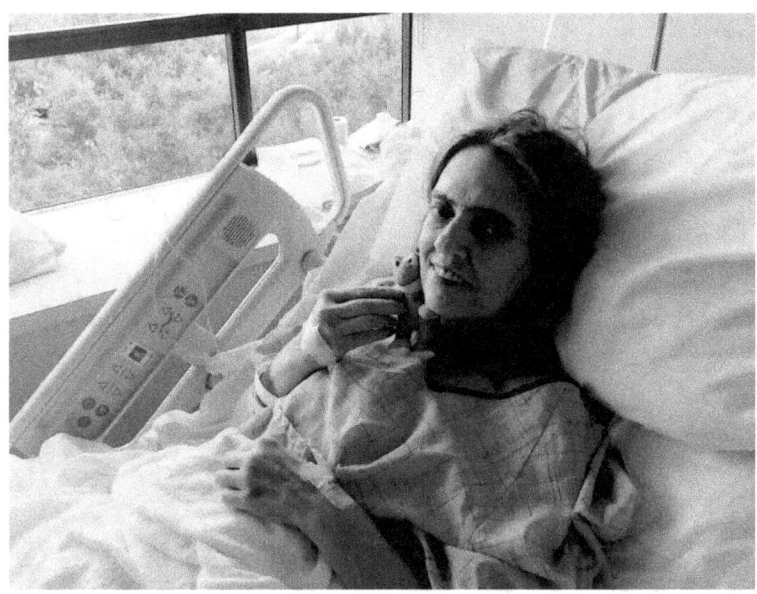

Here's the love of my life the second
time back at the hospital, in her
yellow hospital gown, always funny,
always hopeful.

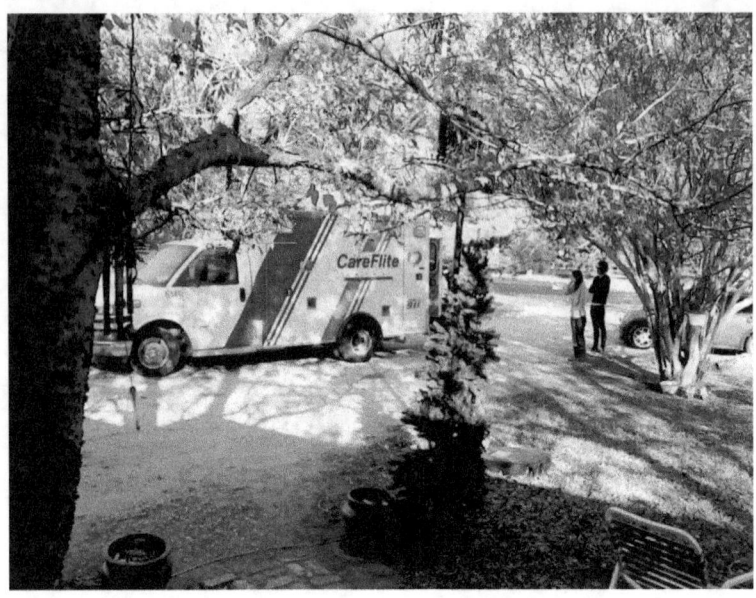

This is the day that the hospital gave
Patricia a ride home Kristie and her
friend follow the ambulance back to
the house.

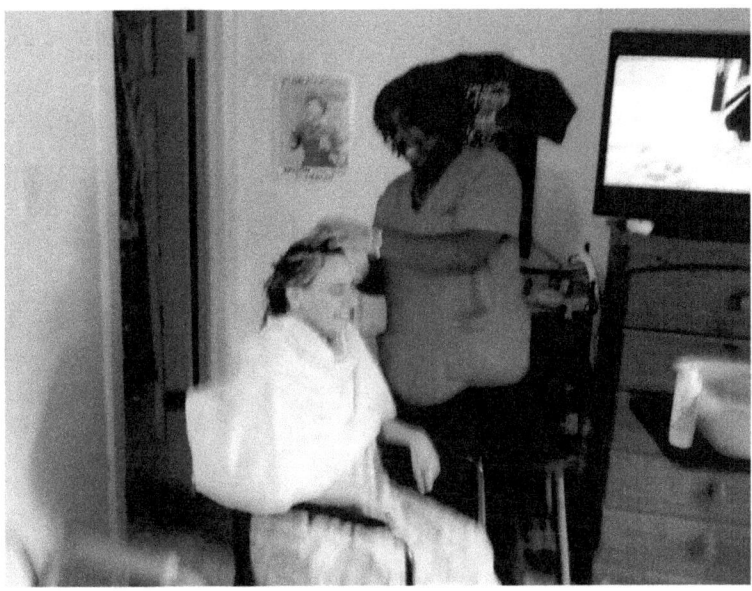

Here's Ms. Rita washing the hospital stay out of Patricia's hair on the first day with hospice, they become such great friends.

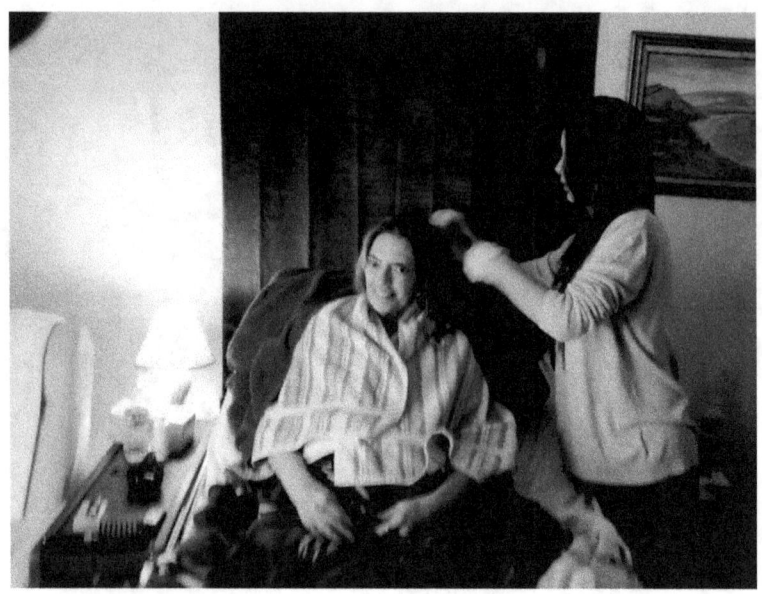

Here's Kristie coloring her mother's hair. What a fun day!!!

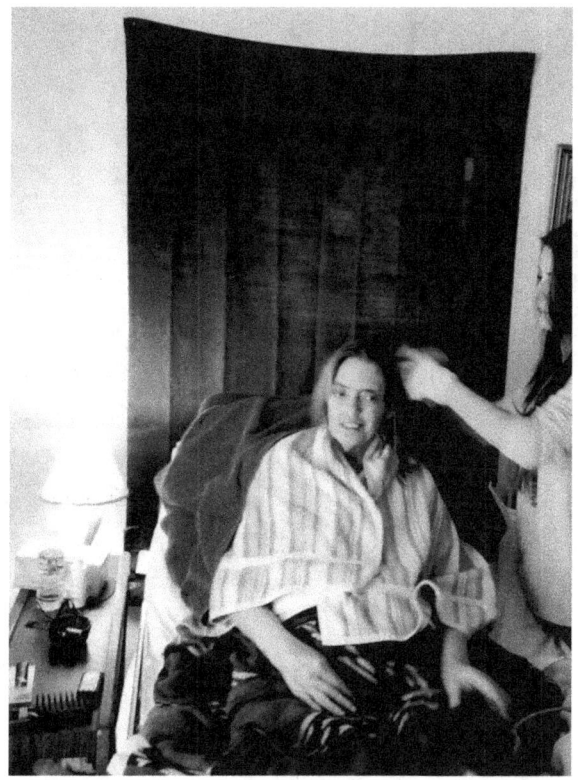

Patricia is enjoying spending time with Kristie.

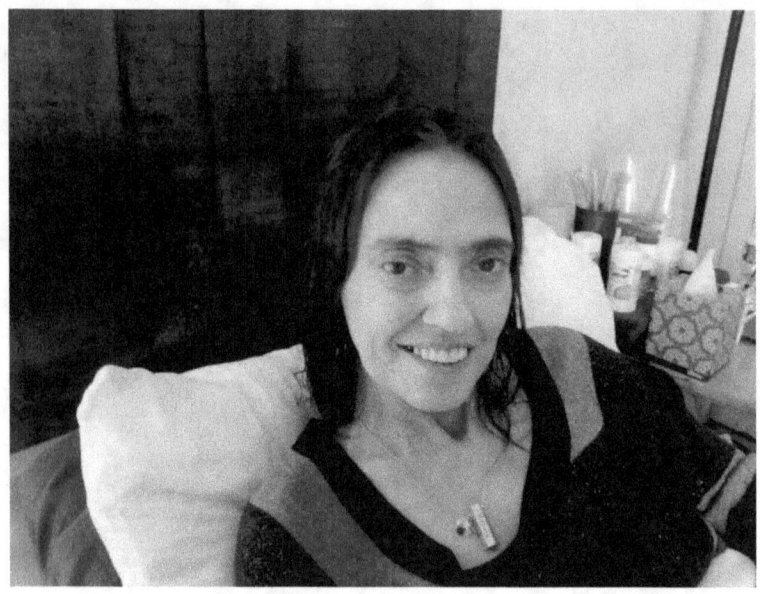

Patricia was very happy with her new hair color.

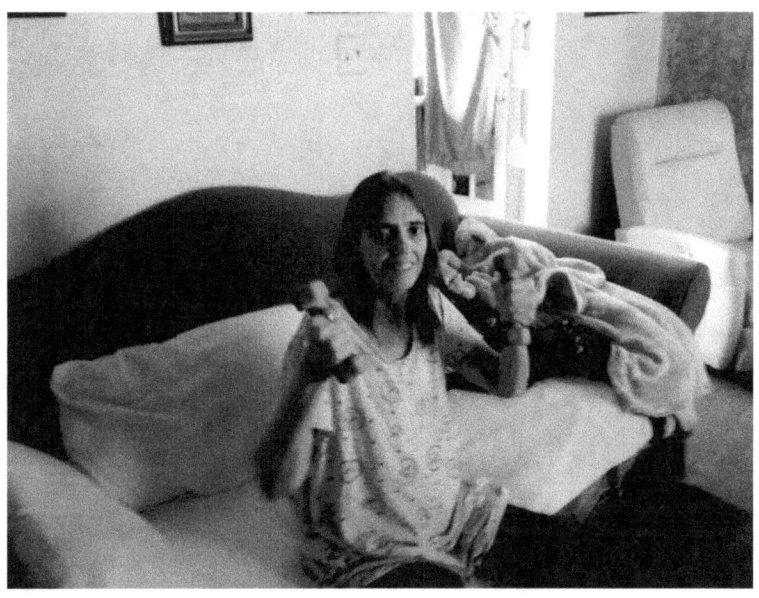

Here's my girl pumping iron always
in it to win it! Patricia was always
showing so much strength in her
hope and faith. God love her.

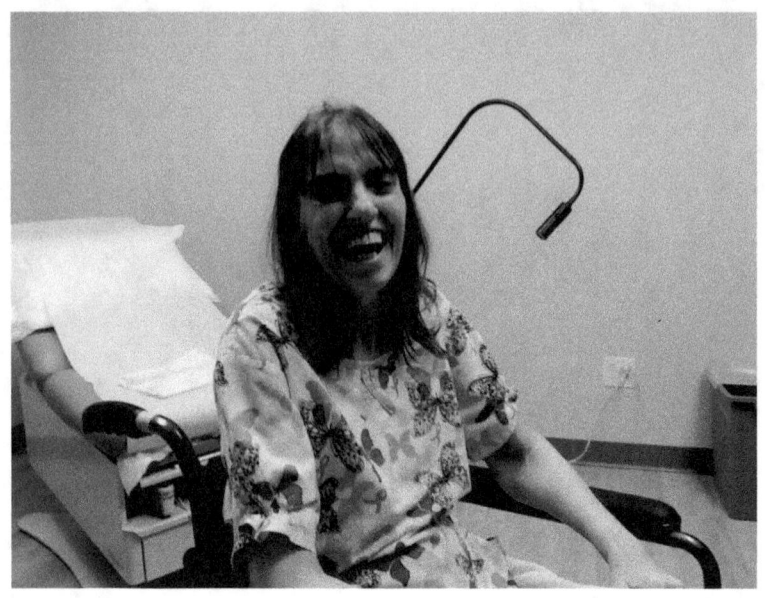

This was a happy day for Patricia. She was off of hospice and the radiation doctor gives some good news.

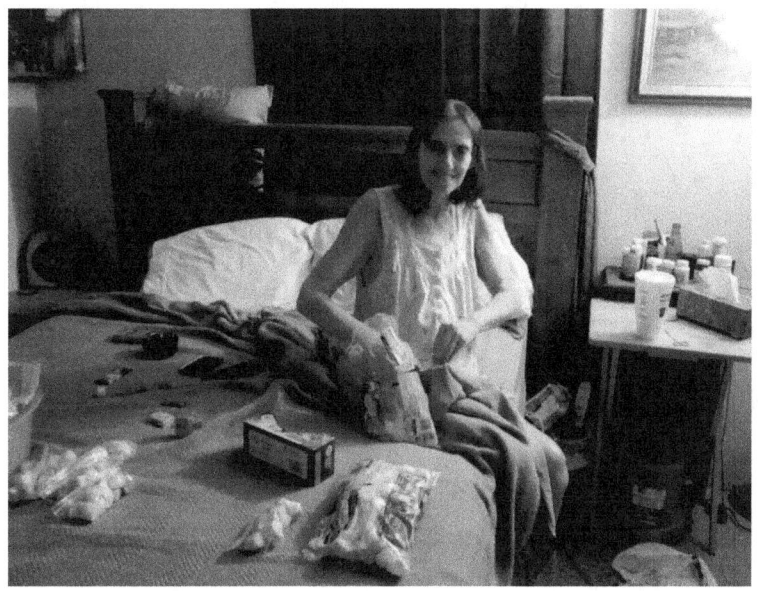

There's Patricia on Easter making
stuff up for Easter baskets. She was
happy to have the bed back in our
room set up.

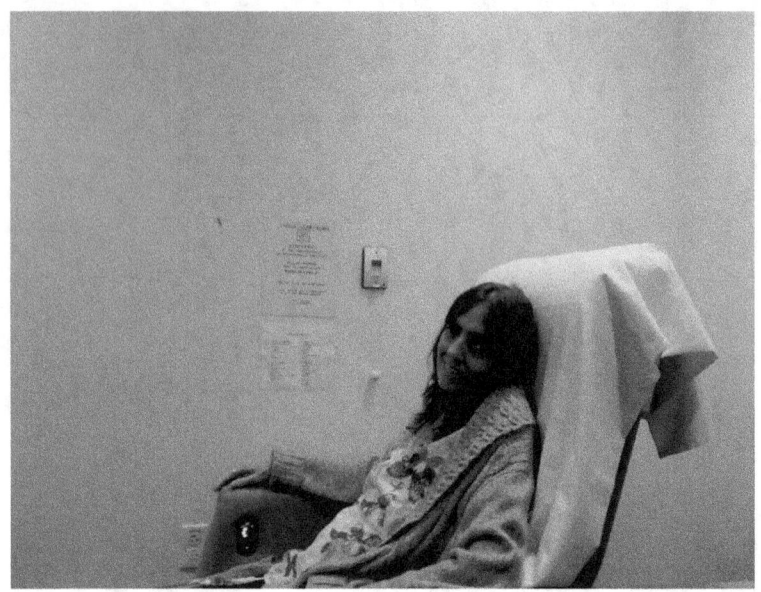

Here is Patricia at Baylor Hospital on
the day of her PET scan being so
positive and this picture is also the
one I used for the cover of the book
Patricia's voice taken 04/15/2015

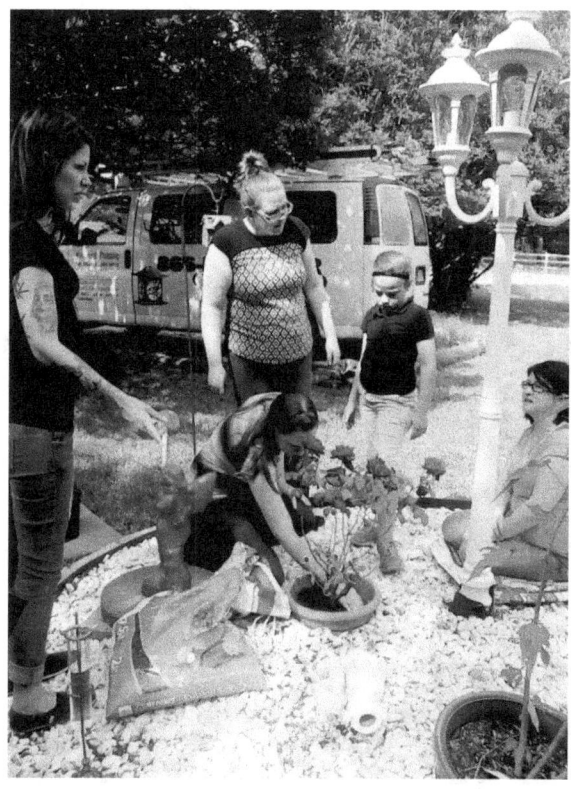

Here's the rosebush. We all picked out two plants in Patricia's honor for her memorial. We have set it up in the rock garden with the lamppost. We called Christian Dior and one of the granddaughters to help.

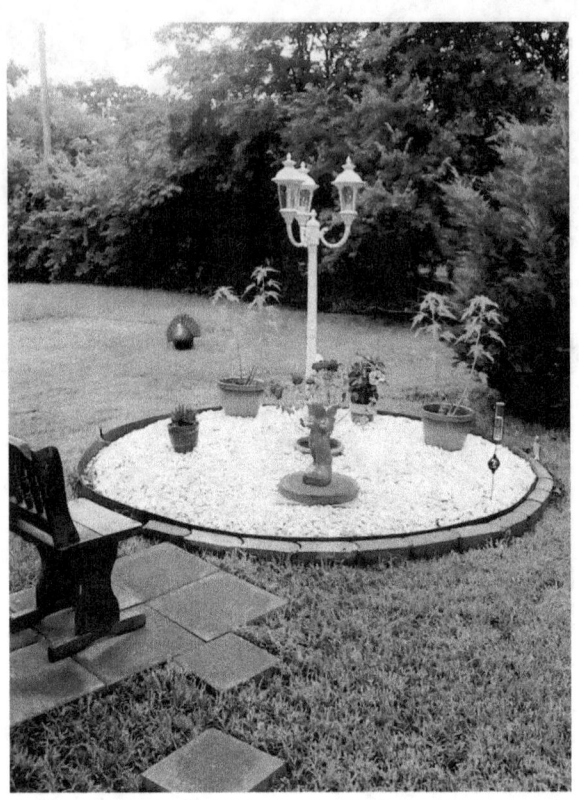

This is a beautiful picture of the rock garden with the lamppost taken on the day of Patricia's memorial service. Friday, 05/29/2015

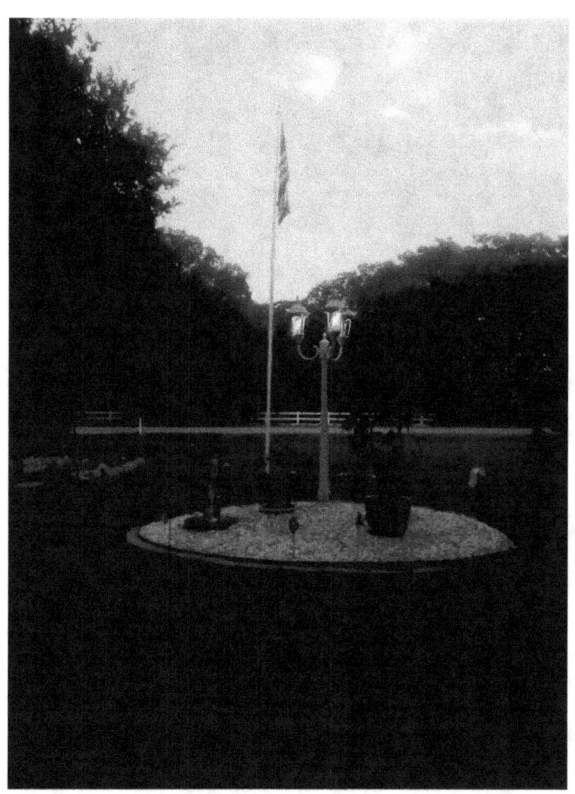

I will be sure to keep the lamppost of hope and faith on to shine every night in Patricia's honor.

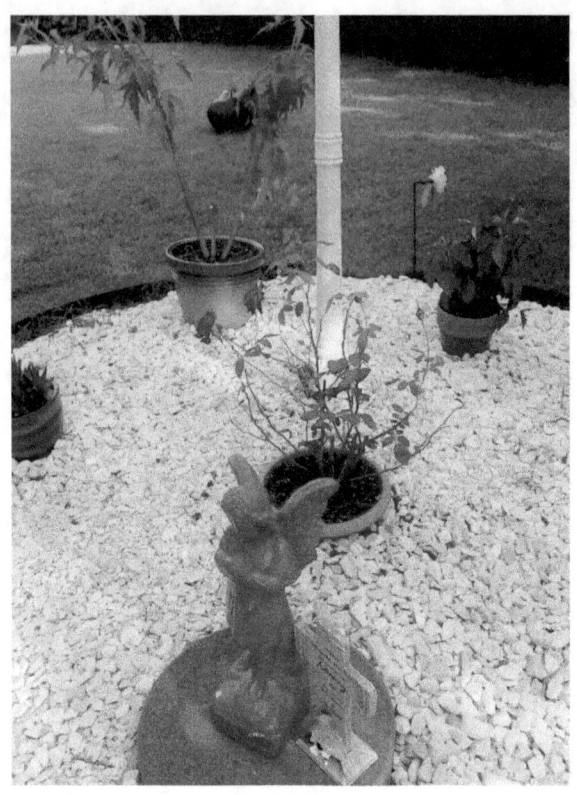

This is Patricia's Angel of hope, peace
and love. Never let your heart
Hardened!

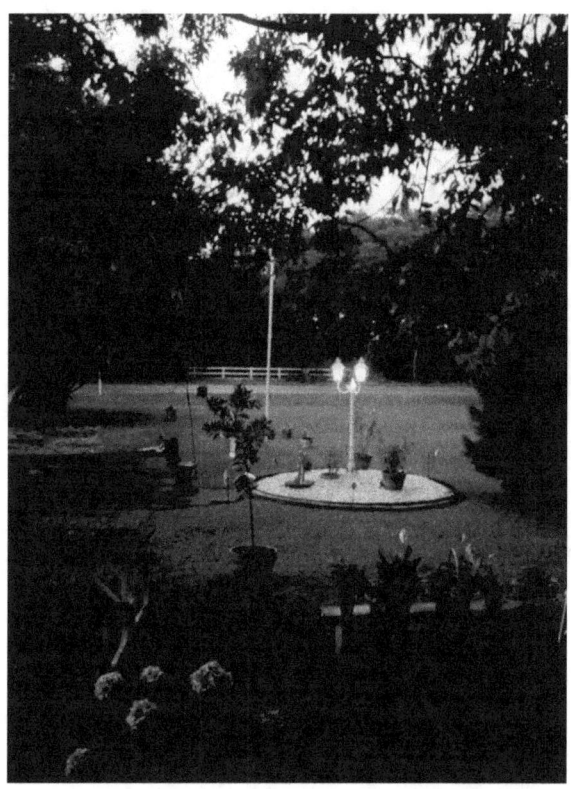

This is the view from off the front
deck of the house.

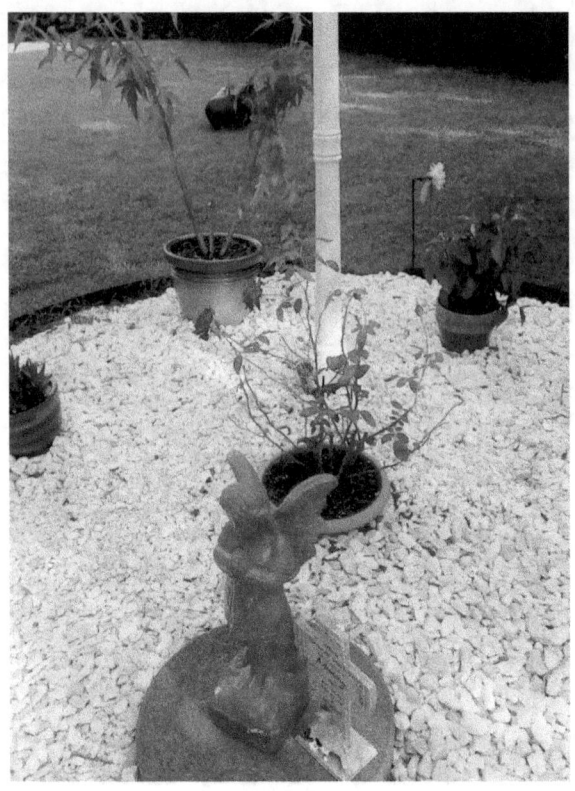

The cross there says, "When the one
you love becomes a memory, the
memory becomes a treasure."
Patricia, I got this and your voice will
be continually heard!

www.ingramcontent.com/pod-product-compliance
Lightning Source LLC
Chambersburg PA
CBHW060616290526
45793CB00001B/42